PARENTS AS PARTNERS IN CHILD THERAPY

CREATIVE ARTS AND PLAY THERAPY
Cathy A. Malchiodi and David A. Crenshaw, Series Editors

This series highlights action-oriented therapeutic approaches that utilize art, play, music, dance/movement, drama, and related modalities. Emphasizing current best practices and research, experienced practitioners show how creative arts and play therapies can be integrated into overall treatment for individuals of all ages. Books in the series provide richly illustrated guidelines and techniques for addressing trauma, attachment problems, and other psychological difficulties, as well as for supporting resilience and self-regulation.

Creative Arts and Play Therapy for Attachment Problems
Cathy A. Malchiodi and David A. Crenshaw, Editors

Play Therapy:
A Comprehensive Guide to Theory and Practice
David A. Crenshaw and Anne L. Stewart, Editors

Creative Interventions with Traumatized Children,
Second Edition
Cathy A. Malchiodi, Editor

Music Therapy Handbook
Barbara L. Wheeler, Editor

Play Therapy Interventions to Enhance Resilience
David A. Crenshaw, Robert Brooks, and Sam Goldstein, Editors

What to Do When Children Clam Up in Psychotherapy:
Interventions to Facilitate Communication
Cathy A. Malchiodi and David A. Crenshaw, Editors

Doing Play Therapy:
From Building the Relationship to Facilitating Change
Terry Kottman and Kristin K. Meany-Walen

Using Music in Child and Adolescent Psychotherapy
Laura E. Beer and Jacqueline C. Birnbaum

Parents as Partners in Child Therapy:
A Clinician's Guide
Paris Goodyear-Brown

Parents as Partners
in Child Therapy

A CLINICIAN'S GUIDE

PARIS GOODYEAR-BROWN

Series Editors' Note by
David A. Crenshaw and Cathy A. Malchiodi

THE GUILFORD PRESS
New York   London

Printed in the United States of America

This book is printed on acid-free paper.

Last digit is print number: 9   8   7   6   5   4   3   2

The author has checked with sources believed to be reliable in her efforts to provide information
that is complete and generally in accord with the standards of practice that are accepted at the
time of publication. However, in view of the possibility of human error or changes in behavioral,
mental health, or medical sciences, neither the author, nor the editors and publisher, nor any
other party who has been involved in the preparation or publication of this work warrants that
the information contained herein is in every respect accurate or complete, and they are not
responsible for any errors or omissions or the results obtained from the use of such information.
Readers are encouraged to confirm the information contained in this book with other sources.

Library of Congress Cataloging-in-Publication data

Names: Goodyear-Brown, Paris, author.
Title: Parents as partners in child therapy : a clinician's guide / Paris
    Goodyear-Brown.
Description: New York : The Guilford Press, [2021] | Includes
    bibliographical references and index. |
Identifiers: LCCN 2020050327 | ISBN 9781462545063 (paperback) | ISBN
    9781462545070 (hardcover)
Subjects: LCSH: Psychic trauma in children—Treatment. | Play therapy. |
    Parent and child.
Classification: LCC RJ506.P66 G657 2021 | DDC 618.92/891653—dc23
LC record available at https://lccn.loc.gov/2020050327

To my three children, Sam, Madison, and Nicholas,
for teaching me, through all the ruptures and repairs,
the grief and the gratitude,
how to be a parent

To my husband,
for sticking together with me through hard things

And to all the parents who have partnered with me,
for allowing me to walk with their families
through the healing process

You are all my teachers.

About the Author

Paris Goodyear-Brown, LCSW, RPT-S, has been providing clinical care for families in distress for over 25 years. She is the creator of TraumaPlay, a flexibly sequential play therapy model for treating trauma; the founder of the TraumaPlay Institute; Clinical Director of Nurture House; and Adjunct Instructor of Psychiatric Mental Health at Vanderbilt University. Ms. Goodyear-Brown has an international reputation as a dynamic speaker, an innovative clinician, and a prolific author. She is best known for delivering clinically sound, play-based interventions focused on trauma recovery, attachment repair, and anxiety reduction. She is a recipient of the Public Education and Promotion Award from the Association for Play Therapy; has given a TEDx talk on trauma and play therapy; and is the author of multiple books, chapters, and articles related to child therapy. Her mission is to help parents and children delight in each other as they stick together through hard times, and to equip other clinicians to do the same.

Series Editors' Note

As coeditors of the book series Creative Arts and Play Therapy, we are delighted that the series concludes with this much-needed book by Paris Goodyear-Brown. When parents are engaged, involved, and invested in child therapy, it improves outcomes that are data driven. Research clearly supports that parents' involvement in their children's therapy process enhances the results, but the methods for the continuing engagement and investment of this parental involvement are often left unspecified. This book fills the gap in the literature.

The contributing authors and editors in our series represent disciplines ranging from psychology, to art therapy, play therapy, music therapy, drama therapy, Eye Movement Desensitization and Reprocessing (EMDR) therapy, and dance and movement therapy. In this volume, Paris weaves threads from attachment theory research, neurobiological studies, play therapy, parent training, EMDR therapy, trauma research, and trauma-informed treatment into a useful and informative tapestry. She avoids the temptation of trying to conceptualize everything under one theoretical umbrella. The late Salvador Minuchin, when training family therapists, often urged them to look for complexity and to challenge the narrow view of the family when defining the problem. Paris has accomplished this for clinicians who, in turn, will be advising, guiding, and counseling parents.

In our judgment, the therapist's use of self is always a critical variable in the process of therapy. Paris is the ultimate encourager, and she offers by example new hope for defeated and battle-weary families. Parents can be worn down by clashing temperaments, strong personalities in one or more of their children, oppositional attitudes, and argumentative dispositions, without even considering the toll they may bear when trying to foster the growth and development of a child on the autism spectrum or with major psychiatric disorders or other special needs. This book demonstrates how to counteract these negative feelings and behaviors without invalidating parents, and shows them a new, more rewarding path.

The book is more than a creative set of strategies that can be used to engage parents in the therapy process. It provides a comprehensive guide to key components of the therapeutic work with parents, including psychoeducation when that is a primary need. A beautiful account appears at the end of Chapter 3, in which Paris engages a family in making a sand tray together that reveals the various stages of chaos, struggle, and healing in therapy—from defeated, weary soldiers raising a white flag because the resources of the parents were overwhelmed by the issues of their son's violence, to celebrating in the end the combined strength of the parents and their son in successfully overcoming the challenges.

Using various creative modes of expression, the book shows us how to work with parents and families to enable them to overcome their sense of helplessness and powerlessness. Throughout, there are multiple examples of how to skillfully shift the perspective and focus of the parents to help them get "unstuck." In our more than 50 years of working with children and families, we've learned that most parents have good intentions. But when they are stuck in dysfunctional family patterns where negativity reigns, the suffering is enormous. This book provides a respectful and empathetic approach to helping parents. Parents don't need more judgment, but they do need more encouragement.

Another contribution is the introduction of hopeful and liberating language, for example, asking parents to reflect on whether or not their children are in their "Choosing Minds" prior to deciding what parenting path to take. If the child is at the mercy of a hyperreactive amygdala and having a meltdown, no amount of logic, reasoning, or persuasion is going to be effective. Understanding some simple concepts of neuroscience and the "bottom-up" functioning of the developing brain can save parents untold quantities of grief and aggravation. Every day in families across the world, futile power struggles are carried out that lead to sorrow, and many of them repeat the next day or the day after that. Also, since language is so powerful, we love that Paris builds on the work of the late Karyn Purvis and refers to children with histories of trauma and extensive loss as coming from hard places. Using that language instead of "traumatized youth" ultimately emphasizes the context, rather than the individual.

This book also covers reflective attachment work addressing the complexity of the work and skills needed to truly help parents. If a parent is frequently and unpredictably triggered by reminders of their own unresolved trauma, then developing a highly polished set of techniques is likely to be of little avail. We commend the author for resisting the shortcuts so favored in today's world of quick fixes.

The inclusion of the concept of "Window of Tolerance" in Chapter 4 illustrates how it can be integrated into work with parents in a safe manner. In one exercise, the author explains how parents can be encouraged to explain what they need in order to stay in an optimal Window of Tolerance. It is also an effective exercise for any therapist to engage in to pinpoint what he or she needs to be able to achieve and maintain an optimal level of tolerance. Work with children and families can be emotionally taxing and grueling as well as incomparably rewarding. Self-monitoring of our own stress level and our methods of self-care is essential.

In the final chapters, Paris teaches what she calls SOOTHE skills and practical play-based strategies to strengthen the ability of parents to act as soothing partners and to help their children manage powerful emotions and hyperarousal. These strategies, while useful to most children seen in clinical settings, are particularly valuable for children who are highly dysregulated due to trauma. Other crucial topics covered in the later chapters of this book include how to take "delight in the child," an important feature in attachment, bonding, and caregiving, and how to recognize and understand sensory processing difficulties. Paris also guides clinicians in helping parents establish boundaries with their children. Following the lead of Daniel Siegel's *Parenting from the Inside Out*, she encourages clinicians to explore with parents their "hooks," or the behaviors of their children that trigger strong emotional reactions in them. Throughout their book, the author offers clinicians numerous exercises, handouts, and activities to explore these hooks in creative and playful ways.

We are confident that both new and advanced practitioners will find many valuable approaches and strategies in *Parents as Partners in Child Therapy: A Clinician's Guide*. These innovative and effective methods clearly illuminate the author's years of experience as a skillful therapist and provide a roadmap to helping clinicians and parents discover partnerships to improve children's lives.

DAVID A. CRENSHAW, PhD
CATHY A. MALCHIODI, PhD

Preface

This book has evolved as an answer to questions from clinicians who train with me: How and when do we bring parents into the treatment process with their children? My answer, after 25 years of practice, is as follows: We want to include parents as partners in every instance in which it is clinically sound to do so. The science seems clear enough; inviting parents into the therapeutic process can maximize treatment gains, but how and when in a course of treatment? This is where the art of therapy is required, the nuanced responding of curious and compassionate clinicians who can shift fluidly between work with various parts of the system as they ask the question "What can the system hold?" I am the creator of a treatment model called TraumaPlay, a flexibly sequential play therapy model for treating trauma and attachment disturbances. The TraumaPlay therapist functions in three roles with families: Safe Boss, Storykeeper, and Nurturer (all terms that will be unpacked in this text). We are always working to help parents grow into these roles over the course of treatment. In most cases, helping parents shift their paradigms about a child's big behaviors, expand their ability to hold hard stories, support their skills in co-regulating the child with more attunement, and delighting in their child more frequently maximizes treatment gains. In some cases, caregivers need much supportive work for themselves prior to being able to step into these roles in their child's treatment. In the saddest of cases, a caregiver is simply unable or unwilling to participate in a helpful way in the child's therapy. A core TraumaPlay value is following the need of the child. As we apply this to the family, we are working to follow the need of the system. This requires a responsiveness that can flexibly move between individual sessions with children, individual sessions with parents, dyadic sessions with one parent and a child, and potentially full family sessions. While there is broad-reaching support in the literature for the incorporation of parents into the therapeutic work of children with a wide range of mental health concerns, there is overwhelming research support for the enhanced efficacy of treatment when we include parents in treatment specific to complex trauma and attachment disturbance.

We have a treatment center called Nurture House in Franklin, Tennessee. It is a single-family dwelling that has been refurbished to offer a multitude of safe spaces to help families and children heal. Attached to Nurture House is the TraumaPlay Institute. We train clinicians on-site, doing practicums in the treatment rooms of Nurture House; we provide online continuing education; and we offer trainings all over the world. The TraumaPlay model is an umbrella of evidence-informed treatment components, each supported by a series of interventions, both directive and nondirective, that are developmentally sensitive and help families move toward healing when hard things have happened. The TraumaPlay treatment flowchart is shown in Figure P.1.

Although this flowchart looks linear, we offer our trainees a graphic that frames the goals within a pinball machine (see Figure P.2), because the fluid nature of the model relies on the clinician making nuanced choices that follow the child's need along the way. While the TraumaPlay model has been written about in depth elsewhere (Goodyear-Brown, 2010, 2019), this volume is focused on how we help parents become partners in their child's therapeutic healing. Notice that the TraumaPlay component focused on soothing the physiology has two substreams. The first involves enhancing self-regulation for the child, but the second arm involves enhancing the role of parents as soothing partners. Chapter 5 will focus specifically on the set of SOOTHE strategies that we offer to parents as we help them increase their ability to co-regulate their children. The other area in which a parent plays a key part in treatment is as a child's Storykeeper. Clinicians understand that we are only in a child's life for a period of time and we want to create coherent narratives of hard things within the family. Parents are welcomed and incorporated into any or all of the key components of treatment. Part of the clinician's ongoing role with the family is gauging when and if parents are ready to be involved in treatment. Are they big enough containers to hold the story? Are they regulated themselves? Will the parent add to the corrective emotional experience of a child in any given session? When are collateral sessions best, and when are conjoint sessions the most effective way to bring delight back to the system? We provide a combination of *in vivo* session work with parents and children together, parent coaching and reflection sessions for parents themselves, and sessions with just the child or teen.

All of these questions are addressed in supervision, and, at Nurture House, parents are pretty frequently and fluidly moving in and out of sessions with their children. We also do an enormous amount of parent coaching sessions and sessions that involve Reflective Attachment Work (RAW) with parents on their own. Our team sees families in every kind of distress. We see many adoptive families in which parents are raising children with complex trauma histories. We see parents who are trying to figure out the best way to parent an anxious child, a child of divorce, a child who struggles with impulsivity and focus. While specific skills sets may need

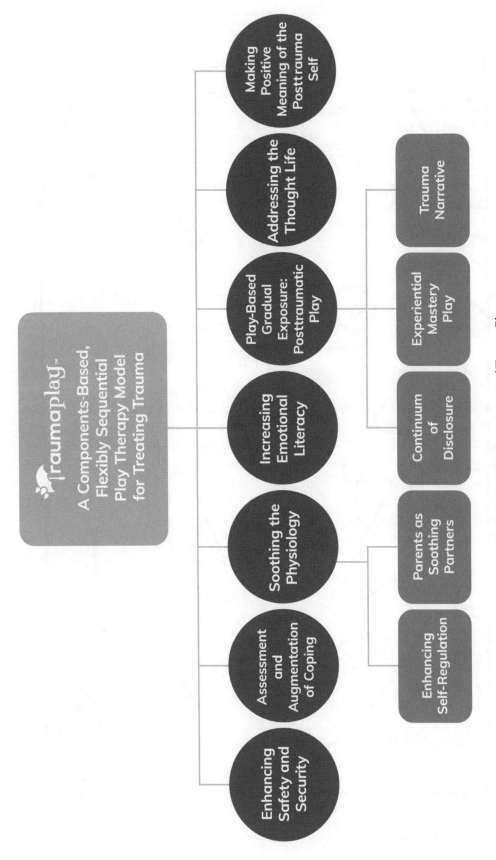

FIGURE P.1. Key Components of TraumaPlay.

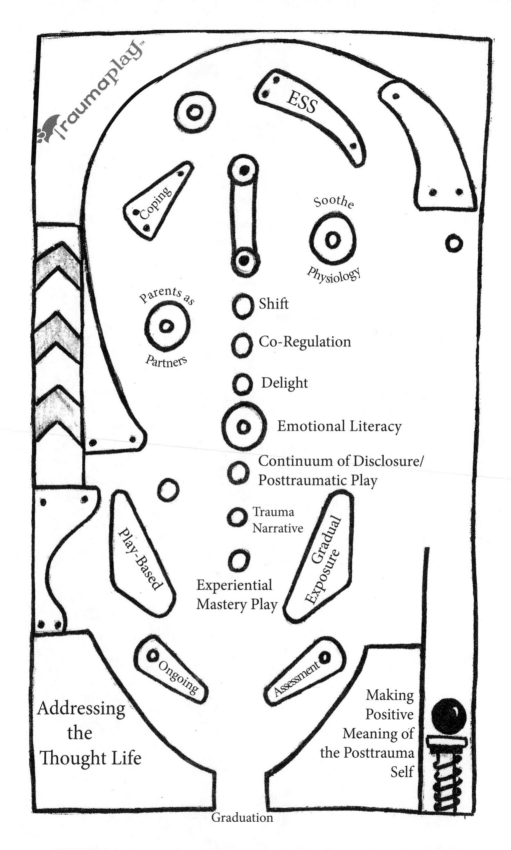

FIGURE P.2. TraumaPlay Mapping Tool: Fluidly Following the Child's Need.

to be enhanced differently in some of these cases, we have found that the essence of the paradigm shift we want to help parents make is that as they stick together with their kids, they can do hard things. Parents have the hardest job in the world . . . and the most rewarding one. Helping parents see their essential value to the tiny humans in their care is one of my greatest joys. Parents often need someone to believe in them, to help them breathe in their power to help their children heal and grow. It is our great privilege to walk with them along the way.

How to Use This Book

Throughout the book, I will highlight important paradigm shifts we help parents to make. Handouts that will be immediately useful to you in sessions will be offered. Case examples will also be woven throughout. I have attempted to use gender-neutral or gender-inclusive language throughout the book in an effort to avoid bias toward a particular sex or social gender. Also, I have attempted to use gender-neutral language in the handouts themselves, in order to recognize that a variation exists in who may be mothering, fathering, or providing daily care for a child from a hard place.

In most of our parent training work, we include in-session prop-based exercises that encourage both left and right hemispheric engagement, supported by handouts that parents can take with them. These may serve as transitional objects from the therapeutic space in which the parent has started experiencing some success— some shared delight and enjoyable moments with their child—to the much more difficult home environment.

The use of concrete tools, such as handouts, to support therapeutic homework for parents serves several purposes. In this case, they offer the following benefits:

1. Exercises designed for parents help communicate that they are a really important part of creating change in the system.
2. The exercises offered through the handouts help support the clinician's work with parents all along the way.
3. Some handouts are meant to provide psychoeducation and important paradigm shifts.
4. Some of the handouts help parents to practice new adaptive skills sets in a supported way, encouraging small doses of positive practice that can generalize to other situations.
5. Some of the handouts are geared toward supporting corrective emotional experiences as parents reflect on their own attachment history with a deeply curious and compassionate clinician.
6. They offer a level of accountability outside the session for response patterns practiced in sessions.
7. They set the stage for the therapist's celebration of a parent's hard work.

Parents are the most important influence in the lives of their young children, and if they steward that influence well, they remain important voices in their child's development over a lifetime. It is critical that we begin working with parents from a place of compassion, acknowledging the impossibility of being perfectly regulated, perfectly kind, perfectly _____ (insert whatever word a parent may see as ideal parenting). It will help us to assign positive intentionality to parents all along the way. It is my deep and abiding hope that as we help parents stretch their containment capacities, become more nuanced co-regulators, and hold their children's hard stories with compassion, we will be doing our small part to build cultures of kindness family by family, community by community, until kindness infuses our global community.

Contents

CHAPTER 1

Helping Parents Grow
GENTLY SHIFTING PARADIGMS

Parenting is the hardest job in the world. To be a parent is to have your heart living outside your body. I am a mother of three. At the time of this writing, my children are 18 (Sam), 14 (Madison), and 10 (Nicholas). I want so much to protect my children from all hurt . . . and sometimes the hurt is coming from me. Facing this hard truth can often be painful for parents and is best supported and cushioned by the help of a compassionate and playful clinician who is committed to sticking together with a family through trying times. This book is meant to equip clinicians to help parents make the paradigm shifts needed to minimize parenting behaviors that polarize parents and children, while maximizing the marvelous power that parents have to be Safe Bosses, Storykeepers, and co-regulators for their children. Parents are the most powerful influences in the lives of their young children, yet parents often don't understand their own power, or even believe that they have any. I have had hulking 250-pound dads, professional football players, describe their feeling of absolute helplessness in the face of their 3-year-old's tantrums. I have had high-powered moms, wildly successful in their chosen fields, admit their bewilderment in the face of their 10-year-old daughter's silent treatment. Therapists who work with dysregulated children balance two roles in their work with parents. We are empowering parents to hear and see their children more fully while bringing the best parts of themselves to their interactions with their children. Parents are superheroes, each in their own right. The vast majority of parents want to show up for their children, to use their power to support their children, but some simply don't know how. Parents tend to parent in the same way that they were parented or in direct opposition to the way they were parented (especially in cases where a parent may have been abused or punished harshly as a child). This may leave little natural room for reflection on their current practices, but can invite opportunities for growth if we make it our goal to join with as much care and kindness with the parent as we join with the child. So much of our work with parents is parallel process work, providing corrective emotional experiences, powerful paradigm shifts, and *in vivo* moments of having parents and children delight in one another again. Perhaps it would be most clear to describe my thinking about systems work, particularly for families in distress, as a Cascade of Care—pouring into the parent what we want the parent to pour into the child.

If this is the goal, then we must interact with parents in ways that communicate our bigger, stronger, wiser, kind presence to them. There are times where parents really need some parenting themselves, and while this statement is never meant to diminish a parent's grown-up status or responsibility and capability as a caregiver, it is meant to help us remember that even parents need nurture, need to have their confusion and insecurity acknowledged and held, need to have a safe space to look at their parenting patterns and their family of origin issues as they relate to current parenting practices. Parents also need to interact with someone who willingly celebrates their growth and all the tiny victories along the way in this impossible job called parenting.

To work systemically is no small undertaking and requires us to maintain a duality of care, remaining curious about the experience of both parent and child all along the treatment continuum. From the first moments of an intake with parents, when they might characterize their child's behaviors in ways that feel diminutive to us, or might ascribe motives for the behaviors they see that are not the motives we would ascribe, it helps us to try and understand their day-to-day experience of the child. In the TraumaPlay model (Goodyear-Brown, 2010, 2019), we offer an assessment phase that allows us to meet with the parents without the child present for the intake. We have two sessions, whenever possible, immediately following the intake that are dyadic assessment sessions. In this way, the child is introduced to Nurture House in a way that is depathologized. We call these Nurture House Dyadic Assessments (NHDAs), and they include some observation of the dyad in the lobby, how they negotiate getting to the treatment room, child-led playtime, parent-led playtime, parent-led cleanup time, and some tasks on cards that help us to see how the parent provides certain dimensions of parenting (structure, engagement, nurture, and challenge), while simultaneously observing how the child receives each of these dimensions (Goodyear-Brown, 2019). Only then do we meet with the child independently for two to three sessions. During each of these sessions, we engage in child-led play, working to enter the child's world, for part of the session. The other half of the session is spent completing specific play-based assessments that help us to conceptualize the child's current emotional literacy and coping repertoire, and to invite their perceptions of the family dynamics. Then we have a parent feedback session, again without the child, and share our synthesized observations. We also share our treatment plan based on this systemic case conceptualization.

Although there are many environments in which clinicians may not have the luxury of an extended assessment phase, many of the tools in this book have been developed based on the systemic needs of families observed during these assessments. These tools will be helpful in the working phase regardless of how your intake is structured. When I share our model with others, some clinicians ask if our clients become impatient with the assessment process. Certainly that happens occasionally, but by and large our families feel held and perceive that we are genuinely trying to understand the dynamics of their specific family before we give recommendations. Here's the other thing to keep in mind: Each of the tasks we ask parents and children to complete in the first phase of treatment is not just an assessment; each is assessment as intervention. Asking a parent and child to pause and interact together in proscribed ways that are unusual to them in their day-to-day interactions (such as asking them to engage in physically nurturing behaviors, or asking them to tell a story about a hard thing that happened) is a form of intervening. Both the parent and the child experience and then reflect on aspects of their relationship that they do not have the time, energy, or inclination to engage in regularly.

My husband and I, and our three children, all box together at a place called Title Boxing. It is really intense exercise, and more fun to do together than alone, but it generates a ton of dirty, smelly wrist wraps. One laundry day, I decided to put all the wraps into a delicates bag (so they didn't get wrapped around the center of the washer). I thought I was being pretty smart; I couldn't have been more wrong. When I unzipped the bag to pull out the wraps, I couldn't find the beginning or the end of any of them. They were hopelessly tangled (see Figure 1.1). As I worked for

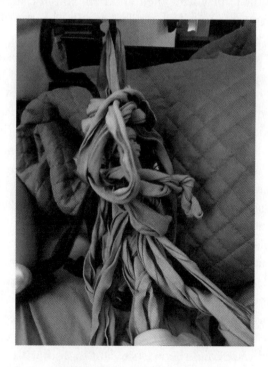

FIGURE 1.1. All Tangled Up.

the next 30 minutes to untangle them, I thought, this is exactly what we are doing with children and families. We must contemplate both questions: What is it like to be the child of this parent? What is it like to be the parent of this child? Simultaneously. Teasing apart how the entanglements have occurred, how the stress has built up in the system, and how to begin untangling things is at the crux of family work. Helping both parents and children to feel seen, valued, and delighted in is critical. Helping both parent and child take responsibility for their parts of the problem areas in family life, communicate their needs more effectively, and receive challenges to maladaptive or dysfunctional patterns of responding are equally important tasks. Clinicians who engage in parent–child and or family systems work can often feel as if they are spinning several plates at once.

Information Overload

By the time parents come to my office, they have usually read the first chapter of five to ten separate parenting books, have implemented several strategies for some period of time, and are still feeling adrift and alone. Clinicians who are grounded in interpersonal neurobiology (IPNB) understand that relationship, as defined here by connection, attunement, shared mindsight, and co-regulation, is the primary change agent for any client in our care. As a play therapist, I build all of these dimensions with children through play and expressive arts work with children. I help parents learn how to play with their children, and in the process the connections between the two deepen. TraumaPlay, our flexibly sequential play therapy approach for treating traumatized children, invites parents to be present at any point in treatment where it meets the need of the child to have the parent present. TraumaPlay maps a series of key components, and one of these is specific to enhancing the role of parents as soothing partners. TraumaPlay practitioners consider it a win anytime a parent shifts a paradigm in a way that is helpful for the child's healing and anytime the parent can hold the story of the hard thing that happened. The parent's readiness to participate in any work meant to help bring coherence to the trauma narrative of the child is being carefully and constantly assessed during treatment, and parents are held (metaphorically) by the therapist as they grow into a big enough container for the story. We will discuss this further in Chapter 9, on strengthening the Storykeeper.

Throughout this book, we will be using the word *parent* to stand for any reliable, committed grown-up caregiver in a child's life. Foster and adoptive parents, kinship care providers, grandmothers raising their grandchildren, and a myriad of other Safe Bosses are included in our description of "parent." At Nurture House, our child and family treatment center in Franklin, Tennessee, if the client is a child, the parent becomes an integral, if extended, part of the client system. Some might say, "Hold on!" Are child therapists meant to work with parents on the deep intrapsychic conflicts with which they wrestle? Of course not . . . except for when we are. Are child therapists meant to help parents trace back their roots of anger to their childhoods? Of course not . . . except for when we are. Are child therapists meant to help parents narrate their own traumas? Of course not . . . except for when we are. Being a systems-oriented, attachment-focused, trauma-informed child therapist is messy work. We are not meant to replace the parent's own personal therapy process, but the age-old adage "If Momma ain't happy, ain't nobody happy" has been borne out again and again as child therapists have dug in to parent coaching with a mom who needed additional support to become the parent she wanted to be. Part of this process often involves helping parents look at their own attachment histories and their own family of origin patterns, some of which may have been traumagenic.

I find that a titrated process of offering parents a little information mixed with a lot of empathic listening, humor, and curiosity about how the parent's world works allows parents to build safety and security with us. Bits of psychoeducation mixed with lots of coaching, and the modeling of new skills can be more helpful to parents than a fire hose of information. This deeply held belief—that as we walk alongside a family, embodying the heart, knowledge, and skills that we want parents to pour into their children, parents will grow the bottom-up integration of these new ways of being—informs the parallel process approach to therapy outlined in this book. Nurture House has been the crucible in which we have tried out many different ways of meeting parents. Numerous mistakes were made along the way. I cringe when I think about my earliest clinical work: shortly before my own marriage and long before my three children began to teach and temper me. A parent would come in asking about a specific "problem area" with their child. If the parent brought up thumb-sucking, I would flip through my internal filing cabinet, open the generic file on thumb-sucking, and give the parent some strategies. Ugh. I am not sure how seen and heard the parents in my care felt in those first couple of years. Now I know, beyond the shadow of a doubt, that you can only give what you have received. Clinicians are in the privileged position of giving parents experiences they may not have had before. The first and most important way to help a child feel seen and heard is to make sure their parent has the experience of being seen and heard . . . by you. Early in my practice, I would tell parents that they should play with their children more, that they should hug their children more. They would nod and smile, blankly but politely, and go home and continue doing what they had always done. That's because we all need supported practice of new skills and the corrective emotional experiences that grow new capacities.

As you have probably experienced in your own practice, by the time parents bring their children to therapy, they are often exhausted, beaten down, and hopeless. They may be disgusted with the child—and disgusted with themselves. The parents themselves need support, co-regulation, encouragement, and celebration as they move along the treatment continuum with their children. Some parents enter therapy fearing that their own failures have caused their children's problems. Other parents enter therapy fearing that their children are inherently broken. Still other parents enter therapy so bogged down in their own distress that they are unable to see their children's needs and meet them. Still others have standards that are so much higher than the child's developmental level will support. In each of these cases, the therapist may be tempted to dig in and begin offering psychoeducation right away. The thing is that, in most cases, what we want to help grow for a parent is parallel to what we want to grow in the child. An understanding of bottom-up brain development informs our approach to support the bottom-up brain development of the parent in the same ways that we are supporting the bottom-up brain development of the child client. What does this process look like? Parents often enter therapy in either a state of hyperarousal or hypoarousal themselves. In many cases, the first job of the clinician may be to co-regulate the parent in all the ways that we would like the parent to eventually co-regulate their child. We have all had the experience of carefully planning a treatment session full of psychoeducation and the parents show up in crisis. Recognizing the parents' upset in the lobby and shifting the treatment plan from tackling a whole list of psychoeducational strategies to co-regulating the parents begins with meeting them in their distress and becoming their Storykeeper in the same ways that we would like them to meet their children in their distress and become their children's Storykeepers. At Nurture House, this may look as simple as assessing the distress in the lobby, inviting the parents into the treatment room that is also a kitchen, and preparing a warm beverage for the parents while they tell you about their upsetting morning. Often by the time a warm cup of coffee is placed in each parent's hands, that parent feels seen, heard, and supported. The parents become more grounded and regulated than when they arrived, and from a neurobiological standpoint, they may have more access to their thinking brains after this caregiving. While the treatment plan will definitely need tweaking, providing the now regulated parents with a nugget of information and a way to practice implementing a new skill is more valuable than talking at them for a full session when they are unable to really digest what you are offering.

We have the opportunity to begin shifting the parent's paradigm as early as the intake session. Even our language on initial phone calls can make a difference in setting the parent's expectations of treatment, framing the work within a family context, and inching the parent's thinking away from the goal of strictly behavioral change and toward curiosity about the underlying need that is not being met. As early as the intake session, I begin tweaking a parent's judgments of their child's behaviors.

TraumaPlay therapists view themselves as holders of the holder. We recognize that the parent is meant to be the primary holder of their child's big feelings, stories, and physical needs. The ways in which we interact with parents present the opportunity to provide seed to rich soil, sowing into the parent what we want the parent to begin sowing into the child.

Inviting Shifts in Language

One of the ways that we begin to help parents become partners in a child's therapy is to help them shift their way of talking about distress when they observe it in their children. Have you heard these statements during your initial assessment with parents?

> "He's a pathological liar."
> "She only thinks about herself!"
> "He is so manipulative!"

Sound familiar? If you have been practicing long enough, you have had parents come into your office saying each of these very things. When a parent presents with this language, clinicians would be wise to respond as if they are balancing on a tightrope, carefully balancing the need to validate the big feelings underneath the parent's statements while also providing another way to frame the child's behaviors. In essence, we want to meet the parents where they are while beginning to shift their paradigms to those that may be more helpful in truly seeing and co-regulating their children. The tightrope walk can sound something like this:

PARENT: He's a thief—he is stealing at school almost every day!

THERAPIST: Stealing. So, he's bringing things home from school?

PARENT: Yeah, daily.

THERAPIST: How do you handle it?

PARENT: Well, I ask him if he took anything from school today. He says "no," and then later something turns up.

THERAPIST: So, you're asking him and he's not telling the truth? That makes sense to me—he knows he's taken something and direct questions about it probably raise the alarm in his brain. He may just answer a knee-jerk "no!" to avoid getting in trouble.

PARENT: Maybe, but I really am at the point where I can't trust anything he says.

THERAPIST: That sounds pretty yucky. No one wants to distrust their child. It sounds exhausting, having your radar up all the time in case he takes something.

PARENT: (*laughing*) Yeah, well, then I feel guilty. I feel like I spend my life interrogating him. It's making me crazy.

THERAPIST: It's really hard for you to trust him right now, and it may be really hard for him to trust himself.

PARENT (*stopping to think this over for a moment*): Huh, yeah—he seems to feel really bad after—but I think it's because he got in trouble, not because it's wrong.

THERAPIST: So, it brings him distress and it brings you distress. I wonder what would help. It seems like leaving things at school is just too hard for him right now—it's almost like a compulsion and he may need more active help from you to protect him from himself.

PARENT: You think he can't control it?

THERAPIST: I think he may need your brain and heart on board to help him.

PARENT: Well, how do I do that?

THERAPIST: You are his Storykeeper; you keep the history of all the times that he has stolen things. You are the most important person in his life and you see that he is drowning in this behavior. It would help both the behaviors and your overall connection with him if you become the life raft for a period of time.

PARENT: But at his age he should be able to stop on his own.

THERAPIST: "Should" is a powerful word. How do you feel when you think, "He should be able to stop!"?

PARENT: Frustrated . . . pissed really.

THERAPIST: Yeah, "should" means we believe that he can stop and is choosing not to. When we believe our children are deliberately disobeying us, it makes us mad. What if you shift your thinking about his capacity? If you start to think, "It's just too hard for him right now to leave everything at school."

PARENT: Just too hard . . . feels, well, if it were true, he'd need help.

THERAPIST: What if you started assuming that he is going to bring something home every day without your help. That it's a compulsion at this point. And that if you ask direct questions, you will be setting him up to lie on top of stealing. But if you can provide more structure for him, you can sort of save him from himself. What if you go home today and sit down with him and say, "Listen, buddy, I am realizing that it is just too hard for you right now to leave everything at school that belongs at school. So, I'm going to help. We are going to start sticking together at the end of the day. Your teacher and I will figure out a private spot for me to meet you at the end of the day. We will check your backpack and your pockets together before we leave, so if there's anything that needs to be returned, we can do it before we've even left school. No harm, no foul. Just helping your brain learn how to leave things at school. We will do this every day until it's not so hard anymore."

PARENT: Boy, that's a lot of work. I shouldn't have to . . . I know, I know . . . stop "shoulding" yourself.

THERAPIST: (*laughing with parent*) Shoulding ourselves and shoulding our kids. Tricky stuff. How would it feel to say these words: "You're letting me know it's just too hard for you to do on your own right now"?

PARENT: I think I'd like myself better and probably him, too. Clearly what we're doing isn't working.

THERAPIST: Some parents take this basic language and run with it. Others would really prefer a script of some sort to help them structure this kind of conversation. Which would you prefer?

PARENT: The script would be good. I may tweak it, make it my own, though. I might forget the right language to use otherwise.

In the conversation above, the primary treatment goal is to help the parent reset or adjust the bar for behavioral performance at the child's level of development at this present moment in real time. The paradigm shift I am hoping for is that the parent will begin to see the problematic behavior less as something the child is choosing and more as something that the child is growing into. The natural outgrowth of adjusting their internal bar for behavior is that parents have more compassion for their child's developmental process. We validate the parent's feelings and immediately begin to gently challenge the underlying judgment about the child. Another instance in which we begin shifting the paradigm right away is when a parent characterizes their child as manipulative in the initial intake. We will validate how hard it is to have a child who is constantly wanting to be in control, while we also start asking parents to replace the word *manipulative* with the question "What is the underlying need that is not being met yet?" Helping parents learn to say, "I see that this is really too hard for you right now" avoids the use of critical language while reopening the parent's compassion well.

In the scenario just described, if it is difficult for the parent to believe anything the child says, the parent feels unsafe in the relationship, may also feel inept, and the growing edge is trust. If it is hard for the child to tell the truth, the growing edge for the child is *risking* telling the truth. Both parent and child are facing tough issues as they start to renegotiate the relationship. My last goal for these conversations is to reflect to the parents their incredible importance in the process. Parents have superpowers, but by the time they get to treatment, they are often so mired in learned helplessness or disgust at the parenting situation in which they find themselves that they are feeling anything but "super." If we can help them see their incredible value as co-regulators, history keepers, Safe Bosses, and delighters, we will have done our jobs well.

Our culture frequently denigrates parents. Mainstream television programs paint parents as either inept, controlling, too busy to care, out-of-the-loop, or so concerned about being friends with their children that they are unable to fulfill the parenting roles that may make them unpopular with their children (for instance, being the queen bee). When I am sitting with a mom and can support the massive influence she has as she sticks together with her daughter, delighting in her daughter's unique makeup, sharing in her joys, providing correction when needed, and holding her daughter in her hurts, I watch this mom begin to breathe in the knowledge that she is powerful, that she matters. In the Cascade of Care that TraumaPlay therapists deeply value, pouring into this mom is likely to result in her pouring into her daughter differently, showing her daughter that she, too, is powerful and that she matters. The Serenity Prayer says, "Grant me the serenity to accept the things I cannot change, the courage to change the things I can, and the wisdom to know the difference." This hallmark of addiction recovery programs can also be an important mantra for parents, particularly as they work through the process of shifting how they see their role as a parent. I have a plaque, given to me by my children, that offers the definition of a mom. It says, "Mom: Someone who does the work of twenty people for free." This definition was meant to both be a joke and express appreciation for all I do, but if it was the definition I lived by as a mom, I would quickly become bitter and resentful. How the parent defines their own parenting role is the first thing we need to explore when trying to create paradigm shifts in caregivers. So, one of our exercises with parents at Nurture House has to do with helping parents articulate the roles that they currently play with their children.

Teasing Apart Parenting Roles

Last summer, while on a speaking trip in Ireland, my family had the privilege of visiting the Vale of Avoca. We spent hours mesmerized by the processes of the woolen mill. Wool is died into magnificent colors, but the wool is tangled and full of burrs. It is one person's job to separate the strands, individuating them enough so that each can become its own thread (see Figure 1.2).

It's a tedious and time-consuming process, but nothing beautiful can be made until this sifting and sorting work is done. We begin by inviting parents to start a similar intrapersonal process of sifting through their current parenting roles, looking at all the various roles they may play as parents to their child, and setting goals for which roles they would like to discard and which they would like to keep. We then help parents examine *person of the parent* dynamics that might be influencing them to keep over- or underfunctioning in roles that they would like to change. In essence, we begin attempting to untangle the threads of treatment that will be needed to help this family.

One way we start having parents tease apart the roles that they want to fill as parents from the roles that they may currently be playing, for better or worse, includes completing the handout labeled "Possible Roles Parents Play" (see Figure 1.3). This

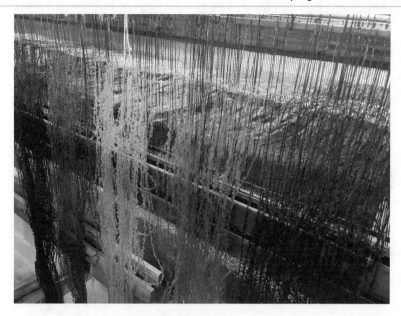

FIGURE 1.2. Teasing Apart.

is a first gentle look at how parents currently define themselves. The parent is given the handout and asked to circle all the roles they fill as a parent. The parent is also prompted to cross out any of the roles that they philosophically can't condone, or believes that a parent should never fill. This usually leads to a rich discussion regarding what the parent in front of you sees as good parenting and bad parenting, and may begin to alert you to strengths in the parent's belief system and places where a paradigm shift might be helpful. One additional offering might be to invite the parent to highlight the roles they would like to grow into.

If we believe, for example, that our role is to protect our children at all costs, we may find it difficult to support their exploration. If a father, for instance, believes he is meant to be a coach, pushing his children to grow and excel, he may have trouble with becoming a safe haven when his children fail or need to be seen and accepted in their weakness. We use the handout to explore the roles that he most identifies with as a parent. Once we have identified these together, we can have a curious conversation about the pros and cons of seeing ourselves in each role.

Returning to the woolen mill, once the burrs have been removed and the threads untangled and smoothed, they are placed in the pattern that the weaver will be using to make the blanket. The pattern repeats as many times as necessary to fulfill the vision of the weaver. Growing healthy children requires engaging in various parenting roles, various patterns of parenting behavior, over and over again. Once the parenting roles have been teased out and the helpful roles have been embraced, parents can begin weaving a rich tapestry of nuanced parenting with their children (see Figure 1.4). Over the course of treatment, child therapists help

Possible Roles Parents Play

Circle your primary parenting roles from the words below.
Put an x through any of the roles that you would never play.
Discuss your most frequent roles with your therapist.
Use a marker to highlight any of the roles
that you would like to grow into.

FRIEND   Detective

MENTOR

Teacher   Cook

Chauffeur

CONFIDANT   BOSS

Slave   Nurse

Servant

MODEL

Nurturer

LIMIT SETTER

Safe Haven

Guide   BOUNDARY ENFORCER

Police Officer   Vision Caster

FIGURE 1.3. Possible Roles Parents Play.

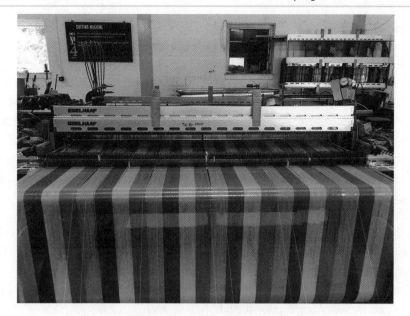

FIGURE 1.4. Creating Patterns.

parents figure out when and how to step into different parenting roles, and, in best-case scenarios, parents leave treatment with a sense of their parenting patterns and the beauty of fully functioning in each of their parenting roles when needed.

I stood in front of the big machine, watching layer after layer of a new blanket be woven, when all of sudden the machinery froze. It didn't screech or bang or slow down, it just abruptly stopped. The sudden silence was deafening. It took a few minutes for one of the technicians to notice the machine had stopped. The worker then came over, squatted down in front of the spools of thread that fed the machine, and saw that one strand had broken. The weaver found both ends and tied them off, and the machine began its rhythmic work once again. The profound parallel between the break in the thread and the ruptures in parent–child attachment relationships fueled a renewed vigor within me to help parents protect the attachment relationships with their children, attuning and repairing them as needed, so that the tapestry of their childhood can continue being lovingly influenced by the parent.

Providing a Cascade of Care

In my experience of families in which trauma plays a central role, parents are exhausted by the time they come into treatment with their child, and they may have even reached the point of being disgusted with their child's behaviors. My goal in the beginning of therapy with parents is simple: to reopen the parents' internal well of compassion for their child.

There are two subgoals to doing this. The first is simply to give the exhausted, disgusted parents large doses of what you want them to give their children. Give the parents corrective emotional experiences and relate to them in the same ways you want them to relate with their children. These include listening deeply to their experiences, hearing the distress, fear, and anger underneath statements like "He's a little monster" or "She's such a jerk" with curiosity and compassion, and without judgment. It is easy for clinicians to begin internally judging the parent who presents in this way and to believe that the problem is the parent. We need to hear and hold the parent's story, the parent's truth, before we can begin to change the story or challenge that truth in any way. If we begin to *talk at* parents as soon as we have identified the first cognitive distortion that they hold, they will shut down. They may smile and nod politely, but real change in the face of defensiveness is unlikely. Clinicians often have lots of intellectual or "head" knowledge that we are hoping to impart to parents, especially to parents who could benefit from paradigm shifts around trauma-informed caregiving. While psychoeducation is a powerful tool, it can only be offered once a parent feels heard, seen, and accepted as they are. A firm foundation of trust and felt safety must be present for deep learning and real change to occur. This comes from listening, psychologically holding, and allowing parents to show the ugliest parts of themselves to us. If we can't meet them first in their story and press into the ugliness, how can we expect them to do this for their children? They are unlikely to be able to look at their own maladaptive coping or the ways in which their own pain and insecurities, their own humanity, are impacting their relationships with their children unless they believe we will stick together with them through it. We call this the "Cascade of Care": giving to the parent what you want them to give to the child.

Narrative Nuance

The second subgoal in reopening the parent's compassion well is especially important when a parent is raising a child with complex trauma. Helping the parent piece together the child's story becomes critical in these cases. A well can only exist in a space where someone has taken the time to dig down, down, down, very deeply into the ground . . . until they hit water . . . until they find the source. By the time parents enter therapy with dysregulated children, they have often lost sight of the source of the behaviors. Layer after layer of boundary violations and other kinds of hard moments are now much like layers of dirt pressed down into hard-packed clay. Clinicians have the job of drilling down through the hardened heart of the parent or the current skewed view the parent may have of the child, in order to help parents see the source of the behaviors. Retelling the child's story—beginning with the child's earliest experiences, those that happened *in utero*—can go a long way in helping to reopen the compassion well for a parent.

I see this dynamic frequently with adoptive parents. They welcomed the child into their home with all the hope in the world. Then the child scribbles with a Sharpie on their couch, which is upsetting, but they push through and move on. Then the child cuts up their biological child's favorite shirt and teaches younger children in the family some inappropriate language. In the end, the number of boundary violations mount inside the parent, creating a sense of helplessness. Helplessness leads to resentment. Resentment leads to either rage or withdrawal of affection. Both the unconditional acceptance of the parent and retelling of the child's story in fresh ways are meant to reopen parents' well of compassion for the child in their care and ultimately lay the groundwork for a paradigm shift. In my mind, helping to create a paradigm shift for a parent is the real win; it's the tie-breaking touchdown of the parent coaching world. A paradigm shift represents a change in both head and heart knowledge and is often encoded by parents neurobiologically in a way that impacts their somatic experiencing, their emotional life, and their thought life.

Usually, fully understanding the child's story also includes understanding the neurophysiological impact that early trauma may have on the developing brain of the child. Chapter 2 will explore ways to help parents understand the science of safety through a neurobiological lens. Figure 1.5 is a handout we use when helping parents to reopen their compassion well. They write either parts of the child's story or mantras that help them to stay engaged and connected, or both, into the lines of the well.

Shame Gets in the Way of Shift

What is the largest barrier to creating paradigm shifts with parents? Shame. What is being described here is another form of parallel process. Parents who have difficulty with their own emotional regulation are often operating from a place of shame. They don't like their anger explosions, they don't like calling their children names, they don't like their own emotional withdrawal from their children, but they feel helpless to change their own behaviors. When we parent out of our shame, we almost always leave destruction in our wake. Brene Brown, one of the foremost researchers on shame, has learned that when she is in shame, she is dangerous to others (Brown, 2015). Understanding this about herself, she has made certain rules for herself: When she is in shame, she doesn't return calls or emails, and she seeks out a person with whom she feels safe to share vulnerably about the experience that engendered the shame. In a parent coaching context, we are the safe person whom parents need to become vulnerable with, but if, when they do so, we begin with "It is not OK to yell at your children" or come from other places of judgment, we will have already lost them. These concepts make sense to us: Meet the parent where he is, try to understand his story, provide unconditional positive regard . . . until we try to apply these maxims in real-life families. Then things become messier.

WRITE THE STATEMENTS, MANTRAS, AND TRUTHS ABOUT YOU AND YOUR CHILD THAT HELP KEEP YOUR COMPASSION WELL FULL.

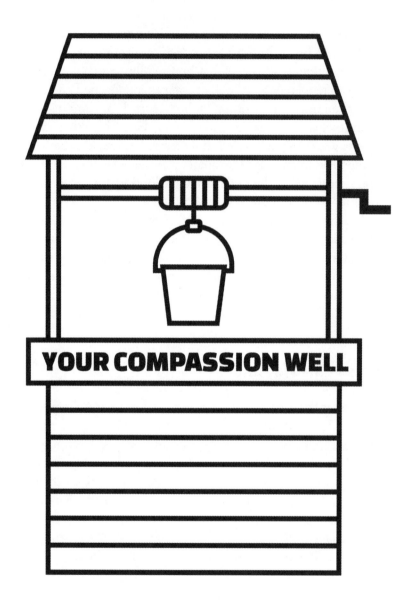

FIGURE 1.5. The Compassion Well.

Transference and countertransference, as well as a basic sense of justice, can quickly trigger child clinicians into a place of defending the child, or even seeing the parent as a monster. I have fallen into this trap myself, almost rupturing my relationship with a new parent beyond repair in the very first session. In one case, a dad (whom I came to admire greatly) described the hour-long rages in which his child would engage. He talked about the bloodcurdling screaming, the many strategies he had tried to help her soothe or interrupt the upset. He confessed that in one of his daughter's intense escalations, out of sheer desperation, he threw a glass of water in her face. He knew he shouldn't have done it, but the act surprised his daughter so much she stopped screaming. He needed me to hold these very intimate shame-centric details of the yuckiest parts of his relationship with his daughter, but I became triggered myself and responded with judgment. My response was "Before I can take you on as a client, I need to know that throwing water in your daughter's face will not happen again. It is incredibly disrespectful and I cannot condone it." I regret that response tremendously, and have wondered with curiosity and compassion about my own origins of hurt that triggered me to so quickly give such a response to this hurting parent. He had already told me that his action wasn't OK. He knew it and was asking for help to understand how to behave differently. Part of what threw me was the incongruence between his affect and the words he spoke. He smiled and laughed a little while telling me about throwing the water. My own fear that the father might again discipline his daughter in this way short-circuited my thinking brain and triggered my own amygdala response. My response created shame in my client and then within myself. Had I been able to remain fully present and grounded, I would have reflected with my face and body the helplessness and desperation he had felt just before throwing the water. Often just an authentic reflection of underlying feeling is enough for the parent to feel seen and heard. I am not saying that we don't set boundaries around safety and practices that might induce shame in the child, but rather that holding the parent's story and shame first establishes a path, a point of connection to facilitate the more important paradigm shifts.

Fortunately, this dad had done a lot of work on himself already and was able to very quickly tell me how my comment affected him. I expressed genuine sorrow at having judged and missed him in that moment, and commented on the multiple ways that he has continued to stick together with his adopted daughter in the face of impossibly destructive behavior. After we had made a repair and this dad knew that I genuinely respected and esteemed him, we could move forward.

"Shoulds" Lead to Shame

We have spent some time on how a parent's shame can get in the way of the parent being able to shift their parenting, because shame shuts down our ability to learn, to stretch our capacities, and to confront ourselves and our patterns with humor and hope. Shame serves no good purpose in a parent's growth process. One of the underlying mechanisms that reinforce a parent's shame is the "shoulds" that person carries around. We all have them—a set of deeply ingrained beliefs about how we should act, what we should feel, what we should think and not think. We have a similarly ingrained set of shoulds about the other people in our lives. For parents, their shoulds are very loud when it comes to the things their parenting partner should think, and feel, and do. The shoulds around what our children should think, and feel, and do are equally loud. Shoulds are judgments and are often unattainable. They refer more to an ideal of perfection than to actual reality.

So, to help parents stop operating out of shame, clinicians need to help them identify the shoulds that are currently guiding the way they judge themselves, their parenting partners, and their children. To this end, we have developed a handout called "The Should Pile" (see Figure 1.6). We give parents 2 minutes, on a timer, to write down as many shoulds as they can about the expectations they have for themselves and other family members. The therapist then helps the parent reflect on these shoulds, how they engender shame when they are not met, and how they are activated in the parent's day-to-day parenting practice. This tool can be especially useful when, for example, a mom brings a COW (Crisis of the Week) to session. Perhaps the child didn't do all their homework, or told a lie. The parent confronted the child and whatever was actually said devolved into a rupture in the relationship. Taking 2 minutes to have the parent reflect on all the shoulds she was juggling—about herself, about her child, and about how other family members should have should not have intervened—can begin to reframe the discussion and shift the mom's focus to internal reflection.

Daniel Siegel, in his groundbreaking book *Parenting from the Inside Out*, talks about the difference between boundary ruptures and toxic ruptures (Siegel & Hartzell, 2013). Boundary ruptures are the moments when a parent and child may feel momentarily disconnected due to a limit being set. If the child has had two ice creams and you have to say "no" to a third, for a moment the child may feel separated from you by that boundary. He has a want and you say "no," but you quickly offer to read a story before bed instead and the child snuggles up with you and feels connected again. Toxic ruptures are those that come from ruptures in the attachment relationship that go unrepaired. Often this is due to the parent's shame. Let's say that a single mom is barely making ends meet. She has a teenage daughter who comes to her on Friday night asking for $20 to go to the movies. Her mom says "no." The daughter becomes disrespectful and accuses her mom of not wanting her to have any fun, and she keeps asking for the $20. Mom, struggling with the shame of not having the money to offer (but unaware that this is her internal struggle), finally explodes and says, "You are a selfish bitch! Go to your room." The teenager storms upstairs, slams the door, and comforts herself by listening to music. The mom storms into her bedroom, slams the door, sits on the edge of her bed and cries. Now she is dealing with the layers of unresolved (and possibly unnamed to self) shame in not having all the resources she would like for her daughter and the new

THE SHOULD PILE

WRITE DOWN AS MANY SHOULDS AS YOU CAN IN 2 MINUTES. DON'T CENSOR YOURSELF!

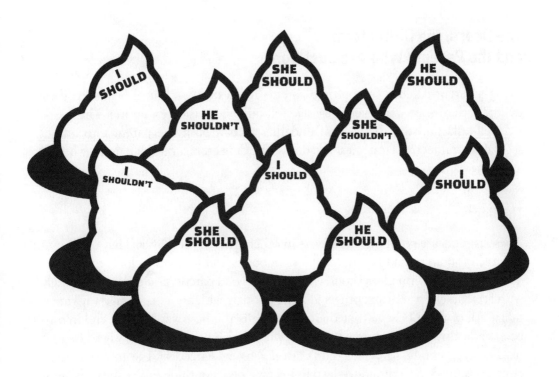

FIGURE 1.6. The Should Pile.

layer of shame at having lost her cool and called her daughter an ugly name. After some time passes, the mom goes back to the kitchen and starts to make dinner, promising herself that she will do better at keeping her cool. An hour later, she calls her daughter down from her room and proposes that they eat dinner in front of the TV. They do so and go to bed with a semiconnected feeling again, but the rupture and Mom's unkind words and actions were never processed, or dealt with. The first time this happens, there is a crack in the foundation of a connected, safe relationship. In parent–child relationships in which unresolved ruptures pile up, the crack becomes a chasm, and eventually neither the parent nor the child know how to get back to an attuned, loving connection.

The Doers, the Deflectors, and the Parents Who Are Just Done

Being a parent is hard. By the time parents reach out for clinical help with their children, they often carry very negative self-talk about their parenting. This negative self-talk, and the shame that underlies it, can push the parent into one of several self-protective strategies: the doers, the deflectors, and the parents who are just done.

The Doers

These parents are often high achievers in other areas of their lives. They came into the role of mom or dad having read lots of books and listened to lots of podcasts. They have pretty firm ideas about what makes a good parent. Some identify strongly with attachment parenting; others identify strongly with an "obey right away" mentality. All of them believe that their approach is the best way to raise children to become healthy, functioning adults who will contribute to society. When the first hard-core parenting strategies didn't "work," as evidenced by the fact that their child continued to be afraid to sleep in his own bed, continued to push the boundaries, continued to display anger or sadness or fear, these parents went in search of alternative answers. They may have a whole stack of parenting books sitting by their bedside. They dive in, get the gist, apply the principles hard core for a period of time, and then move on to the next approach. These parents may have difficulty connecting with their child, as they are seeking strategies for fitting their children into their view of what "healthy" looks like, instead of sitting in relationship with their unique child. The doers will benefit from support in meeting their children where they are. Learning how to simply "be with" their child may be the most important growing edge for these parents. Giving these families protected time to experience 5- to 15-minute doses of child-led play, beginning in the therapy room with the support of the therapist and eventually transferring to the home environment, may be a useful start.

The Deflectors

These are the parents who carry so much shame and negative self-talk that taking responsibility for even minor ruptures with their children feels like admitting to an indictment of their unworthiness. So, they deflect the source of their big emotions onto their children. If you didn't spill the milk, I wouldn't yell. If I didn't have to ask you 700 times to clean your room, I wouldn't end up losing it! The child of a parent who explodes and then blames the explosion on the child learns to accept the blame and to apologize, or begins to move in their own cycle of explosion and blame. In these dyads, the whole culture of the home often needs to be shifted. The first simple treatment goal may be helping each person in the relationship take responsibility for their emotions and actions. Below we outline a tool to structure this process in families.

A few years back, I sat with parents who had brought in their daughter Victoria because she was having rages. Mama did most of the talking during the intake and was clearly more in charge of the home environment than Dad, but both embraced an attachment parenting philosophy. There are many parts of attachment parenting that I as an attachment-based therapist embrace, but these parents had interpreted this parenting philosophy in a way that supported Victoria's complete autonomy. Dad had some trouble with this because he worked from home and his home office, which was the dining room table, had been taken over by Victoria because she "needed" space to build a fort. Victoria had forts in her own room, in the living room, and now in the dining room, but Mama was convinced that it would hurt Victoria's spirit to prioritize one of the grown-up's needs above hers and teach her that her voice was less important than others. Mama's fear of squashing her daughter's developing voice was real and born out of a whole set of her own childhood experiences in which Mama's voice was stolen from her or silenced altogether. So, in such a situation, the question for the clinician becomes: How do we create paradigm shift in a way that helps the parents try new strategies, while keeping the fear of damaging their children in check? First, we have to meet parents where they are. We must work to understand their life experiences and the salient events that have shaped their approach to parenting. To this end, exercises from the Reflective Attachment Work (RAW) part of this book, Chapter 4, will be helpful.

The Parents Who Are Just Done

These parents have exhausted their internal resources and currently cope by simply checking out of the parenting process. Perhaps when the kids get too loud, they intervene to tell them to shush . . . perhaps . . . but otherwise they let the children tend themselves. They don't enforce boundaries around screen time, bedtime, healthy eating, where the children are allowed to go, and so on. These parents are unlikely to seek treatment, but if they do, it is important to figure out what motivates them, as the system is unlikely to change until these parents become inspired with what their parenting role can mean for growing amazing tiny humans.

My Child and Me

When I think about my child, I feel _____.

My child reminds me of _____.

I feel angry when my child won't _____.

I feel sad when my child can't _____.

I feel happy when my child _____.

I feel confused when my child _____.

I feel like a good parent when I _____.

When I think about where my child will be in 10 years, I *think* _____

_____.

When I think about where my child will be in 10 years, I *feel* _____

_____.

I want my child to _____.

The parenting behavior I feel most embarrassed about is _____

_____.

My child needs more _____ from me.

My child loves _____.

My child hates _____.

One thing I love to do with my child is _____.

One thing I hate to do with my child is _____.

I need help to _____ my child.

FIGURE 1.7. My Child and Me.

We can sometimes begin to see how parents are navigating both their emotional reactions to their children and also how they are thinking about their children with the exercise "My Child and Me" (see Figure 1.7). Have your clients fill this out, giving them plenty of time in session to do so, and then process what comes up in their responses.

A Judgment-Free Zone

A couple of years ago, I was walking along a sidewalk in downtown Nashville, holding hands with one of my children. I could tell that heaviness was weighing on him, so I stopped in the middle of the sidewalk and said, "OK. We're gonna start something new in our family. Sometimes kids have things that are really hard to say—they might be afraid they'll get in trouble or hurt their parents' feelings. So every now and then, we will make a Judgment-Free Zone" (see Figure 1.8). "What's a Judgment-Free Zone?" he asked, intrigued. "It's a safe space—while you are in the JFZ, you can say anything at all and you won't get into trouble," I clarified. "Can we use chalk to show where it starts?" he asked. I didn't have chalk on me at the time, so we used some sticks and tall blades of grass to demarcate two squares of the sidewalk as our "say anything" zone. He proceeded to tell me about something that he hadn't before, while standing in those two squares of sidewalk. This intentional boundaried space, paired with both the invitation to share and the assurance that he would not be in trouble, helped him get something off his chest. We continued the walk in a more connected light-hearted way. Since then, there have been a couple of other times when he has said, "I need a Judgment-Free Zone, Mom." I have understood this to mean, both times, that he needed to tell me something but also needed to be assured in advance that we would be OK afterward, that he wouldn't be in trouble.

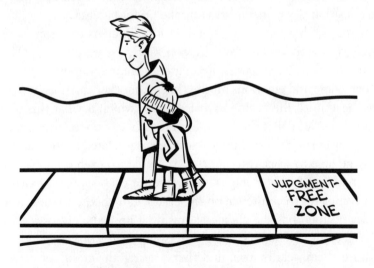

FIGURE 1.8. Judgment-Free Zone.

I have appreciated the prompting in this way, as it has allowed me, both times, to take a deep breath and get into my best, most attentive, most regulated mom self. My hope is that we can provide a similar Judgment-Free Zone for the parents in our care.

Figure 1.9 is a handout for parents that offers them permission to express their negative feelings toward their children. It also helps them to reflect on the feelings of helplessness or confusion that a parent may experience in the face of certain child behaviors. Parents' challenging thoughts and feelings color their interactions with their children and may make it more difficult for a mom or dad's best parenting self to come forth.

The old adage "People need to know that we care before they care what we know" is nowhere more true than in our clinical relationships with parents when they are operating out of shame. I am fourth-generation Italian. My Italian family is given to big emotions. As I have learned the hard way, we are also given to uncensored expression of those emotions. Accompanying these expressions (which might include raised voices, wild gesticulations, curse words flung at others, doors slamming, etc.) is an unspoken belief that such behavior is healthy—letting it all out is the best way to purge difficult emotion. However, children are the most vulnerable members of our society, and they absorb what we say about them like a sponge. It only takes a couple of repetitions of "you idiot" when the child forgets to close the back door, for the child to internalize this talk and begin to call himself an idiot when he makes mistakes. The parent's voice becomes deeply embedded in the child's self-talk. This is problematic. So, what do we do? The question immediately brings to mind actor Bob Newhart's very funny portrayal of a therapist. His mantra was simply "Stop it." Strangely, this was not effective for his clients in TV land. Telling parents just to stop feeling negative feelings toward their children, or telling them to just stop expressing those feelings, rarely results in any useful growth. Parents need to have a place where they can bring their most difficult emotions, fears, disgusts, and hopes to the light, and have them acknowledged by a safe other. It is one of the roles that we as therapists can take on for parents.

To this end, we have created a handout for clinicians that can be paired with an expressive arts activity. Humans are constantly creating a story. We make up stories about all of our experiences, and parents are making up stories about their children's behaviors and emotions all the time. A mother can't begin to change the story in her head until she begins to articulate it, which is what this tool is meant to help parents do. We call it the Judgment-Free Zone: a boundaried space in which parents can project their worst thoughts and feelings related to their children. Some parents may be able to work through this as an *in vivo* exercise. Given a dry-erase board or a chalkboard, the therapist can verbalize each sentence starter out loud. The parent completes the sentence on the board, can choose to show it to the therapist or not, and then has the choice of erasing it immediately, or working around it. There is safety for parents in being able to share their worst thoughts and feelings with you, have them held by you, and then erasing all "proof" of these thoughts. Other parents may prefer to complete the sentences in worksheet form.

Judgment–Free Zone for Parents

My child is so _____

_____ .

When my child screams, I want to _____

_____ .

I can't stand it when my child _____

_____ .

Sometimes I wish _____

_____ .

I feel overwhelmed when my child _____

_____ .

If I could change one thing about my child, I would _____

_____ .

I am disgusted when my child _____

_____ .

I really wish I could _____

_____ .

I don't like myself when I _____

_____ .

FIGURE 1.9. Judgment-Free Zone Parent Worksheet.

Like so many other parent exercises, this one is meant to work on parallel process levels. The therapist becomes the safe container for the parent to share true feelings/thoughts/fears/desperations—even the ugly ones—and the therapist holds them. The parent may then have the experience of relief or of having the feelings/thoughts themselves lose their power or become diffused after the exercise (see Figure 1.9). Our hope is that, after parents complete this exercise on their own, therapists can guide them in a reflective conversation: What was it like to write those things down? What was it like to say them out loud? What was it like to have the thought/feeling heard by another? Through this conversation, parents can shift to a deeper understanding of how holding their child's big feelings in a Judgment-Free Zone may also help defuse the child's big feelings. The feelings and thoughts are there whether we acknowledge them or not. When we name them, we begin to undermine the secret shame that amplifies such feelings and thoughts when we keep them inside.

SuperParents

Once we have confronted the parenting shame that may get in the way of parents creating the paradigm shifts needed for their children to succeed in therapy, we then help parents to set goals for themselves. The TraumaPlay Institute has developed a set of handouts that we share with parents to help them better understand their personal power. We ask them to design the SuperParents they want to become. Inviting parents into the process of setting treatment goals with playfulness often builds bridges with parents. Figure 1.10 is a tool that gives parents a hopeful way to reflect on their current strengths, weaknesses, and the ways in which they want to grow. When parents use their superpowers, they can change the family. For some parents, their desire for X-ray vision parallels their desire to be able to see the need underlying negative behaviors. Parents who use their X-ray vision see straight through the crossed arms and rolling eyeballs to the insecurity or unmet need within the child. What is a parent's superstrength? For some parents, it means being able to carry two toddlers at the same time. For others, it means powering through math homework with your child, even when it takes an hour. I think about Wonder Woman's lasso: When it is thrown around a person, it makes that person tell the truth. In fact, we cannot make children tell the truth, but we can create an atmosphere of felt safety that supports truth telling. We distribute the handout presented in Figure 1.10 to parents and have them play around with designing a SuperParent that represents the parental powers they already have and those they want to grow, and gives some attention to how their own weaknesses get in the way of them being their best selves. Do they need to grow their ability to remain kind when providing correction? Do they need to curb the question monster and grow in their reflective capacity? We have included several symbols around the body: a cape, a mask, a lasso, a shield, a sword. Each of these provides additional strength or power to the superhero, so parents can pick and choose what they need. They may need a cape to cover over their child's mistakes with more grace, or (assuming the cape helps them to fly) to rise above the tantrum their child may be having, maintaining enough distance to see what the next parenting choice could be.

Superheroes all have secret identities, and many of our most beloved superheroes have had early life experiences that inform who they have become: Superman's parents died as his home planet exploded, moments after they had launched him, all alone, into space. The real man behind Batman's mask, Bruce Wayne, watched as both of his parents were murdered in front of him. Some of the parents we treat have experienced traumas equally horrific. All parents grew up with a list of expectations set by their own parents and patterns of relating that are difficult to change, and emotions that may have been warmly welcomed or completely unacceptable within their family of origin. Therapists will explore all of these potential circumstances as parents are gently guided through RAW further into treatment, but this exercise is meant to help parents celebrate the strengths they already have, playfully identify areas of weakness, and set goals for what capacities they want to grow. If, for example, in a parent's family of origin, Mom's mother was cold and withheld affection to communicate her disapproval to her daughter when she did not perform well on a test, there are a variety of ways that this could show up in Mom's current parenting practice. She might name her high expectations of her own daughter as a leftover dysfunctional pattern from her own childhood. In this case, she might perceive these exceptionally high expectations as a weakness and identify them on her SuperParent handout as such. She might have developed this same way of coping with disappointment and be able to reflect on her current tendency to withdraw her affection from her own daughter when an expectation is unmet. On the other hand, she might have decided that she would never withdraw affection from her own daughter. This could show up in a continued connection even during moments when she has to hold her daughter to account; but might also exhibit itself as a tendency not to hold the line on expectations regarding minimum academic standards, and the like, in order to avoid situations that would engender the kind of conflict that might result in her becoming cold with her daughter. I have used this exercise with multiple parents, and some parents have an easier time identifying the most troubling parts of self, seeing themself as "Withdrawing Woman" or "Erupting Man," recognizing that their tendency to withdraw affection or become angry gets in the way of them being the kind of parents they want to be.

When parents start to recognize their own self-protective (and potentially self-sabotaging) behaviors, they can begin intentionally cultivating alternative ways of responding during times of stress. On the handout, the SuperParents' weakness may be a specific child behavior that is triggering. I have had parents identify each of the following: when she rolls her eyes, when he sighs a deep sigh like I'm the dumbest person alive, when she mumbles under her breath, when she is late coming down to get in the car, when I've told him to go to bed and I see his light on a half-hour later, and so on. One triggering behavior that many parents can identify with is when one child hits or hurts another child in the family, especially if that child is younger or weaker than the instigating child. "Erupting Man" labeled himself with this moniker because he would become instantly furious when his 9-year-old son said ugly things to his 7-year-old daughter. His fury, which came out in a roaring voice, scared both of his children and armed their amygdalas so that no useful learning could occur during those moments of correction. He recognized the need to find another way to manage his fury when it came, and after tracing it back to certain triggering behaviors, he was able to practice and implement a redo each time this happened. Moreover, he began requiring his son to make three verbal statements to his sister of qualities he liked about her every time he said something negative to her. The son's behavior was quickly reshaped and, in the meantime, the sister got lots more positive feedback from her brother than she was used to receiving.

The SuperParent's weakness may also be tied to internal processes: their own thought patterns, behavior patterns, or emotions. The mom might identify that when her child's behavior influences her to feel anxious, this feeling is intolerable, so she becomes controlling. The dad might identify that when he sets a clear boundary, he feels confident about his decision for a moment, but then immediately the internal tape of self-doubt starts to play, and he wonders if he was too harsh or critical. Parents begin by completing the "SuperParent Planning Guide" (see Figure 1.10). Figure 1.11 and Figure 1.12 offer male and female versions of the SuperParent.

This chapter sets the stage for the rest of the book. When clinicians embrace the Cascade of Care as a foundational principle in helping parents shift paradigms and grow capacities, we embark on a lifelong mission to continually cultivate compassion and kindness toward parents. We work diligently to assign positive intentionality to parents and to counteract parenting shame as we hold hard vulnerable stories about moments when parents were not in their best parenting self. We understand that modeling containment in this way is necessary for many of the parents that we serve and needs to happen before we ask them to hold their children's hard stories. We look for the Super in each and every parent in our care, while recognizing and embracing their humanity. All of these practices help to build felt safety, as the neuroception of safety is necessary for parents (just as it is for their children) before any neocortex-based learning can occur. As you try out various strategies, tools, or exercises within this book with parents, you may encounter resistance. At the points when resistance seems insurmountable, return to this first chapter and check in around whether or not these foundational ways of being with the parent are present within yourself. Person of the therapist dynamics and continual reflection on our own state of being, on the openness of our own compassion wells, is an integral value held by TraumaPlay therapists and essential for the Cascade of Care to be made manifest in our relationships with parents.

SuperParent Planning Guide

List three superpowers that you believe you need to effectively parent this child. Fill in the blank spaces below and describe a situation in which you need each.

When do you need (insert superpower here) _____ with this child?

_____

_____

When do you need (insert superpower here) _____ with this child?

_____

_____

When do you need (insert superpower here) _____ with this child?

_____

_____

Every parent needs X-ray vision, the ability to see the best self within your child, even when you are angry, disappointed, or afraid. When do you need help really seeing your child?

_____

_____

_____

What is one of your weaknesses?

_____

_____

_____

Secret Origin? Many superheroes have had a struggle in their past that shows up in their present. What's yours?

_____

_____

_____

FIGURE 1.10. SuperParent Planning Guide.

DESIGN THE **SUPERPARENT** YOU WANT TO BECOME.

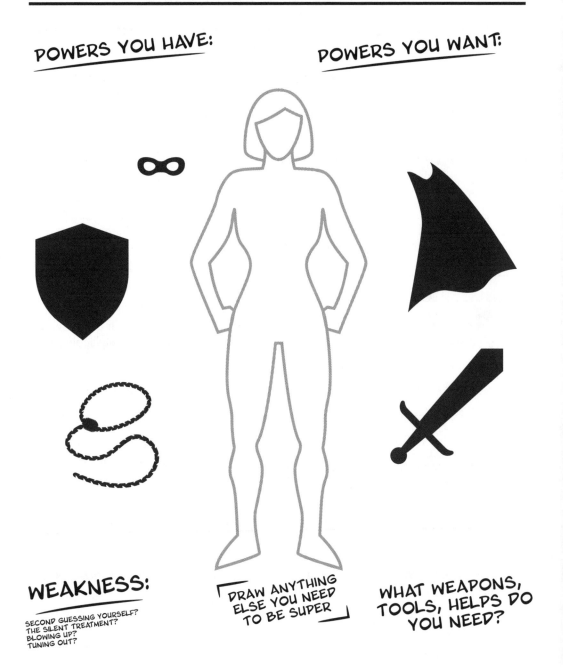

POWERS YOU HAVE:

POWERS YOU WANT:

WEAKNESS:

SECOND GUESSING YOURSELF?
THE SILENT TREATMENT?
BLOWING UP?
TUNING OUT?

DRAW ANYTHING
ELSE YOU NEED
TO BE SUPER

**WHAT WEAPONS,
TOOLS, HELPS DO
YOU NEED?**

FIGURE 1.11. Design the SuperParent You Want to Become (Female).

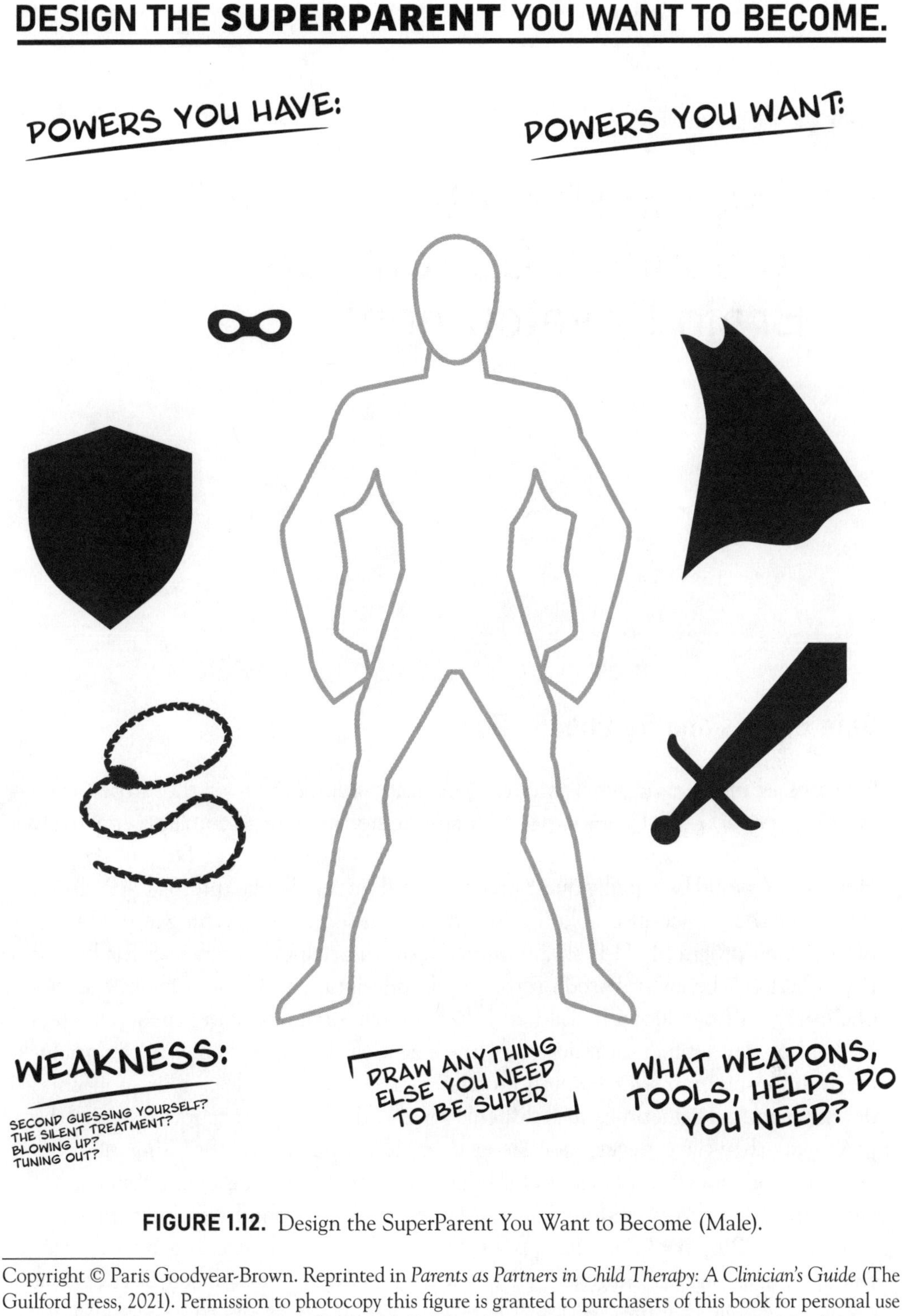

DESIGN THE **SUPERPARENT** YOU WANT TO BECOME.

POWERS YOU HAVE:

POWERS YOU WANT:

WEAKNESS:

SECOND GUESSING YOURSELF?
THE SILENT TREATMENT?
BLOWING UP?
TUNING OUT?

DRAW ANYTHING
ELSE YOU NEED
TO BE SUPER

WHAT WEAPONS,
TOOLS, HELPS DO
YOU NEED?

FIGURE 1.12. Design the SuperParent You Want to Become (Male).

CHAPTER 2

Helping Parents Set the Bar to Support Bottom-Up Brain Development

Safe Bosses and Setting the Bar

Safe Bosses understand what is developmentally appropriate for those they lead. As a supervisor, I would not expect a first-semester intern to be able to effectively map out an entire course of treatment for one of our families at Nurture House. However, it would be equally questionable if I did not challenge interns to do things that make them uncomfortable (for interns, that is usually everything at the beginning of their program). This chapter is given over to helping parents set the bar for their children's behavior based on the child's developmental level. One of the jobs of clinicians who work with children is helping parents understand the parameters for healthy developmental milestones in every area. However, many of the graduate training programs for helping professionals do not include a course on child development, so sometimes it is difficult for the therapist to accurately guide the parent, as they have never been steeped in the principles or the different theorists or developmental arenas of child development. Several excellent resource for clinicians to use in providing knowledge about normal child development exist. Dee Ray's (2016) book, *A Therapist's Guide to Child Development*, is an excellent resource, as is *Ages & Stages: A Parent's Guide to Normal Childhood Development* (Schaefer & DiGeronimo, 2000). It can be soothing to parents to understand, for example, that all children go through periods of equilibrium and disequilibrium. A 3.8-year-old child who is suddenly throwing tantrums and seems disorganized is, in fact, in a stage of normal disequilibrium. The upset is to be expected, but so is the eventual move to reorganization on a new developmental plateau.

Understanding Bottom-Up Brain Development

One way to help parents shift their paradigms regarding developmental expectations of their children is to introduce them to a bit of brain science. Child and family therapists expand our capacity to conceptualize dysregulation more compassionately as we become neurobiologically informed (Hong & Mason, 2016). This same brain-based understanding of behavior can help parents to become more compassionate co-regulators for their children (Hughes & Baylin, 2012). While most clinicians are well aware of bottom-up brain development, most of our parents will need some exposure to this concept. For this purpose, we have developed the graphic in Figure 2.1 to help clinicians introduce parents to the triune brain (MacLean, 1990). One of my favorite explanations comes from the Conscious Discipline model (Bailey, 2015). In this model each part of the triune brain is paired with a guiding question. The reptilian brain stem is always asking the question, "Am I safe?"

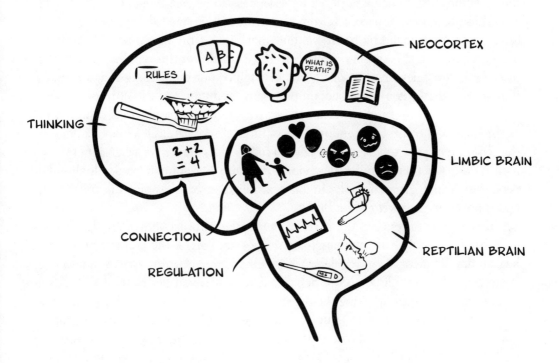

FIGURE 2.1. The Triune Brain.

The limbic brain is always asking the question, "Am I loved?," and the neocortex is always asking the question, "What can I learn from this?" The neocortex, or thinking brain, can only become curious about learning if the other two questions have been answered with resounding yeses (Goodyear-Brown, 2019). Answering these guiding questions with yes requires a child's Safe Bosses to meet the needs of the reptilian brain stem. Clinicians can begin by explaining that the reptilian brain begins to develop first *in utero*, and is responsible for heart rate, respiration, body temperature, and blood pressure. Explain to the parent that this lowest brain region is meant to provide regulation and is responsible for heart rate, respiration, and body temperature—the autonomic processes. The diencephalon, located in the mid-brain (Gaskill & Perry, 2014), manages appetite, sleep, and other arousal regulation patterns. In large part, these lower brain regions set the stage for our sense of felt safety (Perry, 2000). Usually, these processes happen without us even being consciously aware of them. The reptilian brain stem just takes care of these normative functions. On top of the reptilian brain grows the limbic brain, or the feeling brain. This part of our brain is always seeking connection to others. The amygdala alarm, which I have spoken of often in other writings (Goodyear-Brown, 2010, 2019), is located in the limbic brain and is sort of the seat of somatosensory memories as they relate to heightened emotional experiences. So when we see or smell or hear something that is reminiscent of something we saw or smelled or heard during a terrifying or overwhelming event, we may move into a full-blown amygdala alarm reaction based on this sensory input. Specific examples of this will be given as the SOOTHE strategies are unpacked, but it is important for parents to understand that the amygdala is a pretty sloppy processor, and can confuse current sensory input from events and milieus that are not threatening with previous experiences of threat that the child has endured (Gaskill & Perry, 2012; Goleman, 2006). To that end, we are always helping parents to function as detectives when it comes to figuring out whether or not a behavioral response is trauma-related. Finally, the neocortex, which grows over the limbic brain, is referred to as our thinking brain, and is highly underdeveloped at birth.

Developmental expectations, then, must take into account a child's experiences to date, and when traumatic experiences are part of the child's history, the healthy development of our regulation, connection, and learning systems may all be compromised (Perry, 2006, 2009; Schore, 1996, 2001; van der Kolk, 2005). Also, parents can benefit from asking the question, throughout the day-to-day routines of parenting, "Which part of the triune brain am I parenting right now?" For example, if a child is hungry, or tired, the most appropriate parenting response would be to feed the child or put him or her down for a nap. Trying to speak to the thinking brain when the neocortex is offline only ends up in frustration for the parent and the child (Siegel & Bryson, 2011). If the child is feeling lonely, the wise parent will fill the child's love tank with some connected time. Helping parents use the triune brain graphic (see Figure 2.1) can help them provide care with an understanding of what part of the child's brain may need support.

Trauma-Informed Developmental Expectations

Most of the families we see at Nurture House have experienced trauma, and many parents have adopted children who have a complex trauma history. It is important for all parents to understand the ways that their own behaviors can trigger behaviors in their children, but it is critical to parenting a child who comes from a hard place. I wrote briefly about the amygdala above, and provide a whole script for teaching parents about the amygdala alarm when clinicians are going through the TraumaPlay certification process (go to *www.TraumaPlayInstitute.com* for more information). When the amygdala is alarmed, the thinking brain is not available for the parent to reason with. Specific strategies for co-regulating children when they are not in their choosing mind will be shared in Chapter 5.

The Polyvagal Zoo

Another useful way to explain the developmental needs and behavioral responses of traumatized children and teens is through the lens of polyvagal theory. Stephen Porges, a behavioral neuroscientist and professor of psychiatry and human development, is also a pioneer in this field (Porges, 2009, 2011). In 1994, he published something called the "polyvagal theory"—a theory, or body of knowledge, that has given us a more robust and accurate illustration of our triune (three-part) nervous system. His research is also starting to shift the way psychotherapists understand and treat trauma, anxiety, chronic stress, depression, and attention disorders. In order to understand his theory, parents need to know the word *neuroception,* a term that he coined. We neurocept every day. To neurocept just means "to perceive." Porges says that we are constantly scanning our environments for three things: safety, danger, and life-threat, and our bodies respond accordingly. This happens subconsciously, in the most primitive part of our brain. We don't wake up in the morning and consciously say, "Today, I'm going to use the mature parts of my brain to scan all of my environments for safety or danger." Instead, our nervous system does this for us. Inside of our bodies are billions of nerve cells that make up different nerve networks. An important nerve to know about is your "vagus nerve." It is the longest nerve in our bodies, stretching from brain to gut. It's like a walkie-talkie between our brain and our major organs. For example, it tells your lungs to breathe, it controls your heart rate, and it tells our brains to release certain neurotransmitters to calm us down if we get too revved up.

Thanks to the vagus nerve and other nerve networks in the body that connect to the brain, *what happens in the brain affects the body, and what happens to the body affects the brain.* Now, let's turn our focus to the *autonomic nervous system.* Your "parasympathetic system" has two dials or brake systems. One of these systems is called the "social engagement system" (also referred to as the "ventral vagal complex"). This system is activated when you perceive that you are safe. This is our "sweet spot," the system that we want online most of the time. Think about a time when you felt really grounded, in your body, connected in relationships, and calm. In that moment, your ventral vagal complex was dialed up. It's sometimes called the "foot brake" because it helps us (adults) self-regulate. When this system is activated, we feel rested and sufficiently energized. And yet, this is the system that gets hijacked as a result of trauma and chronic stress.

The second brake system is like an emergency brake. It is called the "dorsal vagal complex" (see Figure 2.2). This system is activated in the face of life-threatening danger. This is *not* your fight-or-flight response (we'll get there)—this is your freeze and collapse response. This can look like death-feigning, but can also look like slowing, numbing, shame, and withdrawal. If you've ever felt numbed out or completely shut down, this is because your dorsal vagal system energy is dialed up.

You also have a "sympathetic nervous system" (SNS). This is your gas pedal or your arousal system, the system that is activated when you perceive threat or danger. The keyword here is *perceive*. If you've experienced trauma or live with chronic stress (*not mutually exclusive*), this system is often subconsciously overactivated. Porges says that if trauma remains unresolved or we live with consistently high, untreated anxiety and stress, people develop "faulty neuroception." They may perceive danger in a safe environment or even perceive safety in a truly dangerous environment. Multiple graphic representations of the polyvagal theory exist, as it includes a lot of information to absorb. Parents can feel overwhelmed by the complexity of concepts, as can children. Remember, at a minimum, we have three separate systems: our social engagement system, which is activated when we neurocept safety; our mobilization system, associated with our sympathetic nervous system and activated when we neurocept danger; and our immobilization system, the other end of the spectrum in terms of our parasympathetic response that is activated when we neurocept life-threat. One of the pieces of learning regarding polyvagal theory as it applies to parents is that parents are in a unique position to help their children spend optimal time in their social engagement system. The vagus nerve is attached at the base of the brain with connections to our mouths and ears—we neurocept safety through melodic tones, smiles, and a soft eye gaze as parents' faces communicate delight and safety to their children. When parents speak in harsh tones, grit their teeth, arch their eyebrows in anger, or offer eye contact that is too pointed, the child in their care can be flipped into a mobilization response as the child may begin to neurocept danger. An adopted child who has had previous experiences in which his birth dad yelled at and then slapped him may move directly into immobilization, a life-threat response, when his new adoptive father becomes more intense in his tone.

Since these concepts can be difficult to absorb, we have created a Polyvagal Zoo at Nurture House that we use to help parents and children better understand their neuroception of the world around them. In our graphics, the ventral vagal system (social engagement) is represented by a Very Silly Monkey; the dorsal vagal system, the immobilization response that can look like death-feigning (a tonic, rigid response pattern or collapse, or a floppy, slowed response pattern), is represented by a fainting goat (Dying Very Suddenly) and a sloth (Dying Very Slowly), respectively. The mobilization system that takes the form of fight or flight is represented by an angry bear and a roadrunner, respectively (see Figure 2.2). These playful animals can be used as ways to characterize response patterns that may be seen in parent–child interactions as the clinician begins to learn a family's ways of interacting with one another. Figure 2.3 sets these animals within the context of habitats and can be used to further concretize response patterns of the parent, child, or both.

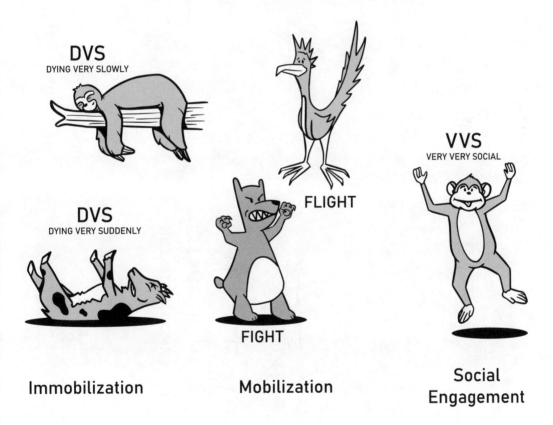

FIGURE 2.2. The Polyvagal Animals.

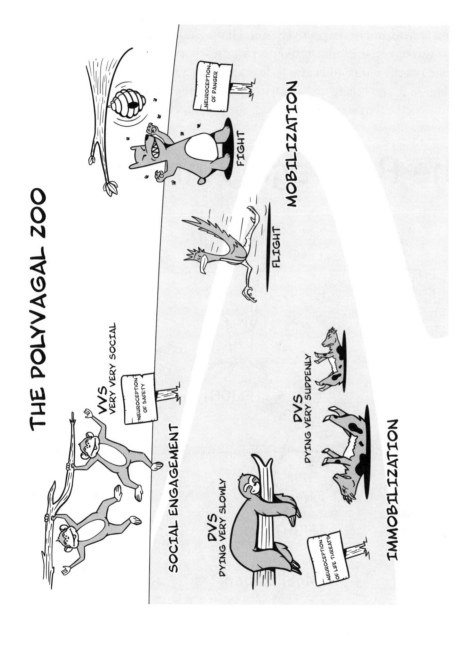

FIGURE 2.3. The Polyvagal Zoo. Adapted from the work of Stephen Porges and Deb Dana.

We complete dyadic assessments with most of the caregivers and their children who come to Nurture House for treatment. Watching the interactions between parents and children in this context can begin to offer a frame for how parent–child interactions increase or decrease regulation in the system. These dyadic assessments can also help clinicians decide which aspects of psychoeducation about our neurophysiology and brain development are needed. If, for example, a child is bouncing endlessly on an exercise ball during his dyadic assessment, and his mother keeps telling him to stop and gets more and more dysregulated herself when the child does not respond by stopping, this parent may benefit from more psychoeducation around regulation and the kinesthetic needs of the reptilian brain.

When Parents Set the Bar Too High

One of the tasks from the Marschak Interaction Method (MIM; Booth & Jernberg, 2010; Martin, Snow, & Sullivan, 2008) is the following: *Adult draws a picture and tells the child to draw one just like mine.* Another of the MIM tasks is *Adult builds a block structure and then says to the child, "Now you build one just like it."* It is not unusual for the parent to have an expectation for the child's drawing ability that is unrealistically high. Sally is a 6-year-old who experienced multiple caregiver disruptions prior to coming into her current home. Mom and Dad are seeking help for the child's hyperactivity, extreme use of force in cases where it is not needed, continual kinetic movement, and rages. As soon as Dad began to draw, Sally asked if he was drawing a house. Dad did not respond and kept drawing. Sally asked a couple of more times and then said, "This is too hard" as she watched her dad's picture

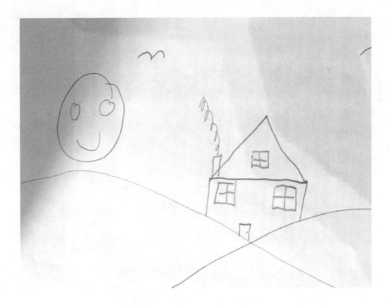

FIGURE 2.4. Dad's Drawing.

develop. Dad said, "You can do it!" And then he added birds, more multipaned windows, hills, a smokestack, and a smiley face (see Figure 2.4). Sally's anxiety, which was already high, as evidenced by her statement that the initial house would be too difficult to draw, put her pen to paper and created the drawing you see in Figure 2.5. It's not hard to perceive the large space between this parent's expectations and the child's ability to approximate that level of performance.

I believe this child was having cortisol releases as she experienced the stress of being asked to attempt something that she already believed was impossible. Dad encouraged her to try and draw it and later expressed his frustration to the therapist, stating that he doesn't understand why Sally refuses to do what Dad wants her to do. Sally is 6 chronologically, but as a result of her developmental trauma disorder, she has significant developmental delays. Her fine motor skills are generally delayed and her drawing abilities similar to those of a toddler.

So, what responses might grow the Safe Boss status of this dad in his daughter's mind and heart? Answering the questions asked helps build Safe Boss status. When Sally asked, "Are you drawing a house?," Dad could have responded with a "yes." Sally would have probably still responded next with "This is too hard." If Dad had said, "Oh honey, this feels really hard for you . . . what's something you think you could copy?" Or, "That seems too hard to you, thanks for letting me know. I'll draw the roof . . . It's really just a triangle, then you can draw it." Dad could have

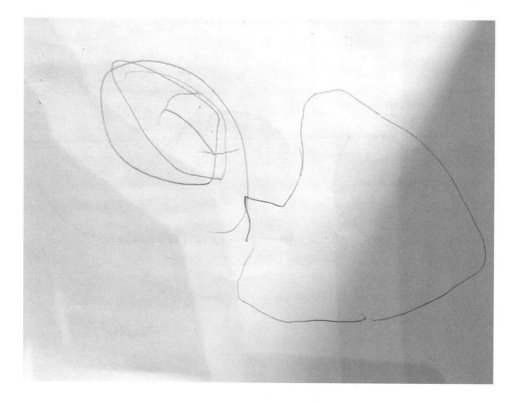

FIGURE 2.5. Sally's Drawing.

stepped the tasks, shape by shape, drawing the triangle, expressing delight when Sally re-created it, and then adding the next shape. Sally could have experienced multiple scaffolding experiences of competence supported by a Safe Boss. More foundationally, it could have been a moment of delight between her and Dad, positively enhancing the attachment bond, the connection to her father, because her father would have been the one to set up the experience of competency. In the same way that teenagers are drawn to people who they think "get them," this little girl would potentially have been drawn into closer emotional safety with her dad if the expectation for the drawing had been developmentally appropriate.

Resetting the Bar

Another powerful benefit of having parents and children together in session is that you can assess how close a parent's expectations are to the developmental bar that is actually reachable for a child. When we were designing the environment for Camp Nurture, a camp we ran for adopted children and their parents several years ago, we knew that we needed a gross motor play environment. Let It Shine gymnastics, a local gymnastics studio that understands dysregulated kids, donated the gymnastics equipment for camp. They hung a rope in the middle of the room, blew up a mountainous-looking slide on one side of the rope, and placed a big, cushioned box-like structure underneath the rope. The children in our camp loved to climb up the side of the slide and perch at the top while a counselor brought the rope to them. They would gather their courage, jump out over empty space while holding onto the rope, swing several times, and drop to the crash mat. Some children were especially fearless, jumping off easily. One camper was the complete opposite, in terms of her readiness to risk swinging on the rope.

Kenyisa, a 9-year-old with low muscle tone, tried multiple times a day to swing. She would climb to the top of the slide, grab hold of the rope knot, and then freeze. We worked with her on other parts of the crash and bump circuit for most of camp, titrating her approach to risk and the resulting competency reward—the surge of dopamine and oxytocin that was supported by the baby-stepped accomplishments. During the last crash and bump interval of the final day, while at least two other campers cheered her on, she was able to risk swinging over to the crash mat. Her less than elegant splat on the crash mat was met with several cheers from other campers and shouts of victory from the staff, who had watched this struggle over the course of camp. The maxim is as true as ever: Those who risk nothing gain nothing. I have embraced this mantra for years and years, but recently I have added onto it: Those who risk nothing gain nothing, and those who risk too much too soon may actually lose ground.

Having a cushy place to land when you fall is a good thing and may encourage you to try again, since the pain of falling isn't so bad, and children will often try again. However, if you crash over and over and over again because the distance between where you started and where you end up is too much, or the bar is set too high, a child's feelings of ineptitude and inadequacy can be reinforced. I recently moved from one form of exercise (kickboxing) to another ("Burn Boot Camp"). We do really hard exercises . . . ones that make me feel like I can't possibly go on. And yet, there is a psychology to the camp's program that always impresses me— just when I think I can't do anymore, that I have reached the end of my capacity, I do more. Sometimes this has to do with someone calling out that there are only 10 seconds left. I always feel as if I can dig back into my internal resources for 10 more seconds. I reset the boundary and count down from 10 as I crank out 10 more burpees, or push-ups, or some other torturous activity. Another strategy employed by the trainer is pairing us up so that my partner is doing sit-ups for as long as it takes me to do 12 tricep dips. Suddenly being teamed with another human, and understanding that my behaviors affect my partner, always push me to do my part with more diligence and more speed than I would have otherwise.

This is what Lev Vygotsky's (Vygotsky & Cole, 1978) zone of proximal development is all about. Vygotsky suggested that a child can achieve a certain level of competence on their own, but can do more with the help of another. His work has informed the question that I ask of parents and teachers: What is the child's growing edge? Implicit in this question is an awareness of what the child is capable of doing on his own and what he can do with the help of another. A great example of this recently surfaced in a dyadic session I had with a mom and her adopted son. When I first met Lily and her son Boe, he was unable to let her help. Many children from hard places have a core belief that they must control everything at all costs, making it difficult for them to ask for help or accept help when they need it. It was a real breakthrough session for this dyad. We had been engaging in nurturing care activities and early narrative rehearsals for the first half of the session. The mom had just reenacted, in the sand tray, the way that she had scooped him up from his sick bed in the hospital and brought him home. She had put the baby in a crib in the sand tray and tucked a blanket around him. Boe watched carefully and then abruptly moved across the playroom to where the foam blocks were kept. He started to build a tower, or some would have called it a wall, between himself and Mom. Mom and I came closer to stay connected, and somewhere in the middle of his building, one block began to teeter like it might fall. Mom gently put her palm up on her side of the wall and stabilized the block. I said aloud, "Mom saw that your tower was in danger of falling and she knew just what to do to help." Boe smiled quietly and continued building. After a few more verbal reflections of Mom's willingness and eagerness to help him, Boe began asking her to help (see Figure 2.6). Eventually, their fingers touched as they stabilized this thing that they were creating together.

One of my great privileges is getting to help parents reset their internal bar for what a child is currently capable of and how we set up the child for success. Parents can underestimate the power of their presence when bringing more of themselves to a situation. More of themselves may be exactly what is needed for a child to feel

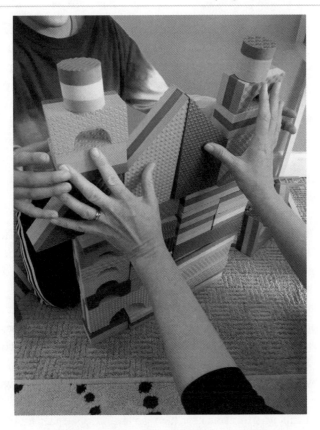

FIGURE 2.6. Mom Supports the Tower.

supported into a place of change. Several years ago, I worked with a mom who had an older biological child who, according to her, was very "easy and well behaved." Mom and Dad wanted to expand their family and couldn't have more children biologically, so they decided to adopt. They adopted a little boy named Claudio from a foreign country, and he was in their home by his second birthday. I did not begin to see the family until Claudio was 6, by which point Mom had become incredibly frustrated with him because he would hoard food, steal money from other family members, and steal things from his friends at school. Each afternoon, when she picked him up at school, she would ask if he had taken anything that didn't belong to him while he was at school. Her hope in asking while still in the car rider's line was to be able to take him back into the school building and return the item before they left the campus, but his answer was always "no." However, at least once a week, when she checked his backpack later on, he would have something inexplicable—for instance, a shiny new eraser that he didn't have money to buy, a cool watch that wasn't his. She would ask him where he got it, and he would always come up with a fantastic lie that made her doubt what she knew, which was that he had taken it. She loved to go to yard sales on Saturday mornings and would take him with her. She would give him a dollar to spend on whatever he wanted, but he often ended up with something in his pocket that was not bought with the dollar. I explained to her that the questions "Did you take something?" and "Where did you get this?" were probably being received as a form of interrogation and would immediately arm his fear-based brain. The fear triggers the lying, and round and round it goes. How can she increase her potency as his primary helper in the zone of proximal development? She can:

1. be his Storykeeper.
2. provide more structure.
3. stick together with him.

Translated into actions, I encouraged her to begin saying, "I know that it is hard for you to keep from taking things from school, so to help make sure you are only taking home the things you came with, we are going to pull into a space after I get you in the car rider's line and we will go through your backpack together, so we both know if there's anything we need to return. This way, you won't be in trouble if you've taken something. We'll just be able to train your brain to give it right back." As she understood that he needed more structure, she also began walking together with him more of the time at yard sales, saying, "I know how hard it is for you to see things you want and not have them, so we will hold hands as we shop and we can figure out together what would be good to buy with your dollar." Eventually, we agreed that even this was too hard for him, so she stopped taking him to yard sales with her at all. She enjoyed the yard sales more, not having to manage the anxiety that he might steal something, and he instead began doing "donuts with Dad" during this time on Saturday mornings.

When parents shift their expectation to "Right now it is likely that he is going to steal sometimes" and see their job as helping the child try out new behaviors in a supported way, much of the parental frustration can be defused. The slight "sting" of consequences or the feeling of shame that may be experienced by securely attached children being caught in a lie, or caught stealing, is quickly mitigated by their underlying rock-solid belief that they are loved and that they are good. Children from hard places do not have this deeply secured understanding that they are loved and good. Therefore, strategies that we might use for creating slight discomfort that leads to growth in our securely attached children only further arms the amygdala of our traumatized children, amplifying their fear and kicking them quickly into a response that is disconnected from care (Purvis, Cross, & Sunshine, 2007; Purvis, Cross, Dansereau, & Parris, 2013). Lying and stealing are both behaviors that hide a part of the true self, the real child, from others: They are both expressions of independence and isolation. We want to be inviting patterns of connected behavior, and this requires noticing problematic behaviors and still delighting in the child while supporting new kinds of interactions.

Most of us value honesty and believe that telling the truth is a noble goal. It is a difficult balance for parents to continue holding up a standard, while fully delighting in their child wherever they might be right now. In my experience, when parents have rigid ideas about right and wrong, when parents say, "In our family, we don't lie," children who have lying all wrapped up with their identity can feel isolated and like bad kids, alone in their badness. I have had adopted children draw themselves as aliens in a foreign land when I ask them to draw a picture of their adoptive family. These children can feel tolerated and even pitied in their own homes. What if we turned this thinking on its head and instead saw these children as remarkable warriors, so clever in the ways that they have learned to survive and get needs met on their own, if we saw it as a great privilege and a gift every time they risk being vulnerable with us, turning to us to get a need met?

Just as inconsistent parenting provides an atmosphere of continual confusion for children, intermittent obedience by children provides similar confusion for parents. Parents don't understand why the child may be able to follow through sometimes but not at other times. However, we only need to look at our own inconsistencies as parents to understand this. Coming full circle to our understandings of bottom-up brain development can help us make more sense of the inconsistent competency that children can manifest, particularly those who had their beginnings in trauma. The cartoon in Figure 2.7 is shared with parents as a humorous way to help them acknowledge that there may be an area of parenting in which their expectation of their child is too high—where they may be setting up their child for failure.

We then offer the parent a separate handout, one that is meant to help parents get really practical about the kinds of expectations they have of their children. We call the expectation "the ask" and offer three heights at which the bar can be set. The lowest bar is the "easy ask." The clinician says to the parent, "What is one expectation that your child can regularly meet?" It might be the child tying her shoes, or brushing her teeth. It might be reading for 30 minutes without help or putting away her laundry without shoving it into a drawer so it wrinkles. We then talk about the "supported ask" and help the parent identify an expectation that the child can meet when he is supported or supervised by the parent. Lastly, we identify the "impossible ask," something that the parent may hope the child can do in an independent way, but that actually will require more developmental time and highly supported practice before it becomes a reliable expectation. From a clinical perspective, it is wise to wait on the use of this handout until you have enough experience with the family system to be able to speak with some authority about the child's developmental capacities in different arenas. When the family is ready, using the handout in Figure 2.8 can structure such a conversation. Have parents write down each of the "asks" in the bars. If you are fortunate enough to have two parents involved in treatment, it is worthwhile to have them share their "asks" with each other in session, as they may disagree about developmental expectations. One may perceive a child as perfectly on par developmentally with a behavioral expectation while the other may believe the same child to be far from ready for the same expectation. In this case, bringing this disparity into the room, naming it overtly,

SETTING THE BAR TOO HIGH

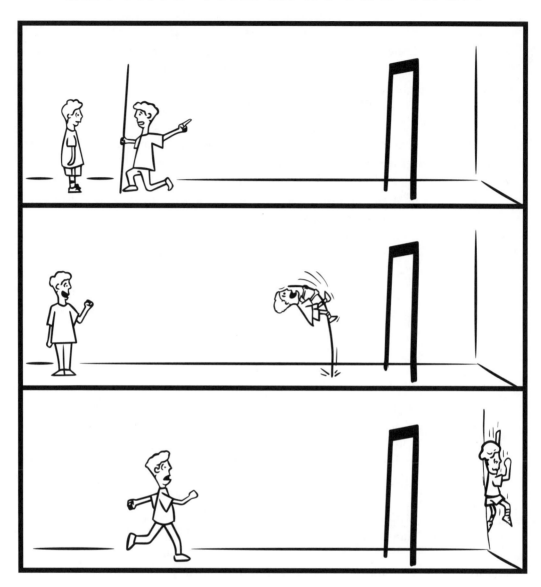

FIGURE 2.7. Setting the Bar Too High.

Setting the Bar for Success

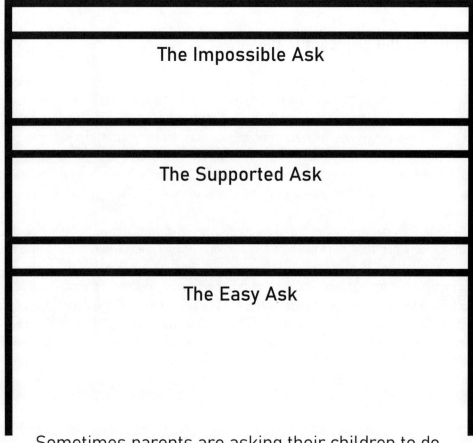

The Impossible Ask

The Supported Ask

The Easy Ask

Sometimes parents are asking their children to do things that they simply aren't capable of doing yet.

In the bottom rung, identify one task you know your child can do on their own. In the second rung, identify one task that your child can do with your help. In the top rung, identify a task that may simply be too hard for your child to do consistently right now.

FIGURE 2.8. Setting the Bar for Success.

and speaking to it from the clinical lens of developmental appropriateness is helpful to the family.

Is This the Hill You Want to Die on?

One final thought about behavior in the context of developmental expectations: Just because a child can complete a given behavior doesn't mean that they will consistently do so. Parents, especially Type A parents, can spend their energies with their children giving instruction after instruction. Pick up your clothes, put your shoes in the closet, say please, brush your teeth. Children are growing creatures, and life is messy. If we want time to embrace the joy, the silliness, and the magic of childhood, we must limit ourselves to the areas of growth that require lots of directions.

Moreover, parents are more likely to get the resulting change in behavior they want to see when they narrow their focus to one or two areas where they would like to see consistency in their child's behavior. Leading parents through the process of setting the bar for success—and identifying the easy ask, the supported ask, and the impossible ask—helps to narrow the field of behaviors that are developmentally appropriate to encourage at this time. We then introduce the handout in Figure 2.9. Parents are encouraged to choose only one . . . or maybe two . . . of the behaviors that we will be working to shift during treatment.

ASK YOURSELF THIS QUESTION:

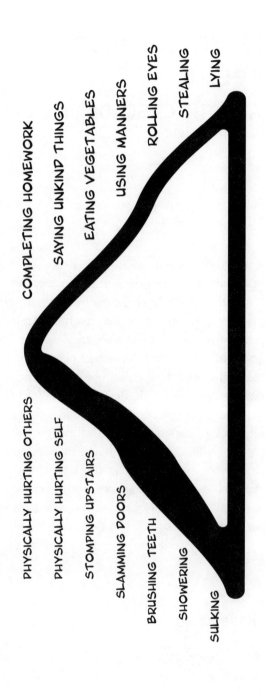

PHYSICALLY HURTING OTHERS
PHYSICALLY HURTING SELF
STOMPING UPSTAIRS
SLAMMING DOORS
BRUSHING TEETH
SHOWERING
SULKING

COMPLETING HOMEWORK
SAYING UNKIND THINGS
EATING VEGETABLES
USING MANNERS
ROLLING EYES
STEALING
LYING

IS THIS THE HILL I WANT TO DIE ON?

CHOOSE ONE _____ . . . OK, MAYBE ONE MORE _____

FIGURE 2.9. Is This the Hill I Want to Die on?

CHAPTER 3

Helping Parents Become Safe Bosses

ATTACHMENT AND THE CASCADE OF CARE

This chapter will focus on how therapists earn the status of a Safe Boss and how we enlist the Safe Bosses in a child's life, such as parents or teachers, to help them approach scary content safely. A discussion of the attachment relationship as foundational to the development of self-soothing is then tackled. We, the grown-ups in children's lives, have profound importance in the neuroception of safety that children perceive, or don't. Embracing our role as a neurobiological anchor is one of the ways in which we embrace our status as a Safe Boss for each child in our care. When children have early experiences of neglect, maltreatment, or institutionaliza-tion, they may have a complete lack of experience with what we would define as a Safe Boss. In fact, the words *safe* and *boss* may be diametrically opposed in the minds of children who have experienced deep hurt at the hands of the adults in their lives. Our team at Nurture House is growing together in how we convey a Safe Boss presence. There are certain universal qualities of a Safe Boss. These are conveyed in the playroom, but they may also need to be conveyed from the first moment that a child is met in the lobby and be expanded upon for parents who care for a hurt child.

Broad Strokes for Safe Boss Roles

I frequently utilize the beautiful graphic produced by the creators of the Circle of Security project (Hoffman, Cooper, Powell, & Benton, 2017; Powell, Cooper, Hoffman, & Marvin, 2007, 2009) with parents when I am providing psychoeduca-tion around attachment. The project's primary graphic consists of two half circles. On the left-hand side of the circle are a pair of hands: one representing the parent as the secure base and associated with the top of the circle, the other representing the parent as the safe haven and associated with the bottom of the circle. When parents are functioning in the role of the secure base, they are supporting their child's exploration. When parents are functioning in the role of safe haven, they are welcoming the child in their distress. While the specific tasks vary based on whether or not the child is on the top or the bottom of the circle, one of the guiding principles at all times is to be "bigger, stronger, wiser, and kind." Being bigger and stronger without having wisdom and kindness leads to a lack of safety for children, but children do need to know that their caregivers are strong enough physically and emotionally to hold their child's big feelings and big behaviors and to set limits when necessary. In essence then, a Safe Boss is a caregiver who can be both a secure base and a safe haven.

Here is the really tricky thing: We are each more comfortable, based on our whole amalgam of life experiences to date (including the attachment patterns within our family of origin, our other relational experiences, our education, and our cultural context), operating on the top of the circle or on the bottom. In other words, each of us is either more comfortable being a secure base and supporting our children's exploration, or we are more comfortable being a safe haven and welcoming them back in their distress. The first question, in the TraumaPlay view of parallel process, is to ask the clinician this: Which side of the circle are you most comfortable with? To be clear, neither side of the circle is better or worse than the other, but if I, as a clinician, am most comfortable supporting my client's exploration, I will only suggest (or even be able to comfortably hold) certain therapeutic interventions with the families in my care. If I, as a clinician, am most comfortable welcoming clients in their distress, I may be great at holding big feelings with clients, but not so great at encouraging them to try things independently and to eventually function in their parenting roles separate from the support of a therapeutic relationship. We find it a valuable exercise to lead parents in an exploration of their roles as a secure base and safe haven, but as play therapists, we offer the exercise cross-hemispherically. Simply put, we don't limit learning to linguistic work with parents about the concepts; we offer mediums for symbolic expression and access the parents' other ways of knowing. In the TraumaPlay model, any of the reflective exercises a therapist asks a caregiver to participate in have already been experienced personally by the therapist in training or supervision. Our belief in parallel process extends throughout Nurture House. We don't want to ask parents to engage in any exercise that we have not experienced ourselves. Moreover, these principles of secure base and safe haven, which originated with John Bowlby, extend far beyond the parent–child relationship. If you are a clinician who doesn't have children yet, identify how you fill either or both of these roles with other family members, colleagues, and friends.

The exercise itself is fairly simple. We unpack both roles, giving examples of both secure base and safe haven behaviors. I begin by painting a picture of a mom and her 3-year-old son who are playing at the park. The preschooler is perched precariously on the second rung of the ladder that leads to the monkey bars. Mom is standing right behind him. As his little body begins to feel the risk of being that far away from the ground, his desire to climb up to the third rung begins to quietly struggle against his desire to stay safe. He looks back over his shoulder at Mom, who holds her hands up in case he needs catching, while smiling encouragingly and saying, "You can do this, buddy! I'm right here if you need me." The preschooler takes a deep breath, struggles up to the next rung of the ladder, and immediately experiences a surge of competency that fills his whole body. Mom was a part of that. Mom was his secure base. She supported his exploration, staying in close physical proximity if he needed her and simultaneously supporting his independence. This is the quintessential scenario that runs through my mind when I think about secure base behaviors in parents. All of us need to have our exploration supported, but at some point children get tired, or hurt, or scared, or sad, or hungry and they come back to their parent. A parent's job at this moment is to welcome the child back in their distress, to be a safe haven. Most parents want to welcome their children back in their distress, but some forms of distress are easier to perceive than others. When a child runs to us crying, with her knee bleeding and asking for a Band-Aid, it is fairly easy for most parents to see the distress and to be a safe haven. However, when an adopted 12-year-old child says, "F___you, you're not my mom. I don't have to listen to you!," it becomes more difficult to perceive the hurt, although this child is equally in distress. This is where the rubber hits the road, being able to get underneath the disrespect or off-putting behavior of the child or teen to see the unmet need of the younger child within. The roles on the top of the circle and the bottom are fairly uniform: In both roles, the grown-up is protecting the child, helping the child, and delighting in the child. The biggest difference between secure base behaviors and safe haven behaviors is one job—*helping children organize their feelings*. When I first experienced this elegantly simplified perspective offered through the synthesized attachment research of the Circle of Security team, I thought "yes"!

At Nurture House, we ask about the parents' current discipline strategies during the intake. When parents tell me that their young son often has screaming tantrums and goes on to explain that they are primarily using a time-out as a discipline strategy, I find it especially useful to go ahead and unpack the child's needs around the circle. As I explain the concept of safe haven, I offer the 5-year-old's meltdown as another form of distress. If we believe that our job when the child is dysregulated in this way is to welcome him back in his distress, and that the primary job while welcoming the child is to help him organize his feelings, it undermines the healthy power of our role to say, "I see that you need help organizing your feelings right now, but I need you to go over there in a time-out and organize your own feelings. When you are done, you can come back to me." Children need more, not less, of us in the times when they are most upset.

Once we have unpacked the two concepts of secure base and safe haven for parents, then we offer each student a paper plate, clay, pipe cleaners, Play-Doh, and markers. When we use a traditional ignore strategy when a child is in the height of their distress, especially when there has been attachment trauma in their life already, we are reinforcing their aloneness, and answering the question, "Will my parent stick together with me when I am showing the worst parts of self?" with a resounding no.

We give the following prompt: Create a symbol to show how you see yourself in the role of a secure base for others. Then create a symbol to show how you see yourself as a safe haven for others. We then invite trainees to break up into small groups and share their experiences of being secure base and safe haven, and to further reflect on this critical question: Which one comes most easily to you? There is no judgment here. All we are asking is for clinicians to become more self-aware of which role they function in most easily, so they can cultivate their presence on the other side of the circle with intentionality. Figure 3.1 shows the clay symbols created by two clinicians who then processed together what each of these roles means to them, how others perceive the clinician in each of these roles, and what all of this means for their growth in being able to hold their clients around the circle. Once clinicians have experienced this exercise themselves, they are often eager to begin using it with the parents of their child clients.

There are no right or wrong symbolic expressions, but the exercise itself invites a level of self-reflection that lends itself to growth and shift. The mother who cheers when her 3-year-old goes to poop in the potty, but become uncomfortable when her 3-year-old clings to her legs as she is trying to leave for work, can be helped by

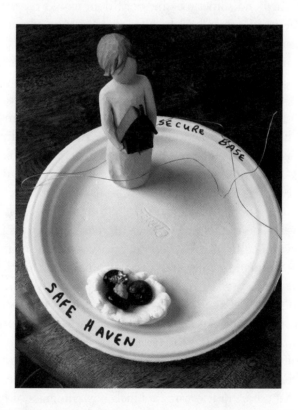

FIGURE 3.1. Symbolic Representation of Secure Base/Safe Haven.

understanding that it is simply easier for her to support her son's exploration than it is to welcome this same child back in his distress. For her, secure base behavior comes more naturally than safe haven behavior. Again, no judgment is associated with this self-reflection, but as awareness increases, parents and clinicians can intentionally grow their ability to function well in the less comfortable role.

Is a Safe Boss Needed?

The simple answer is "yes." Children need to know who is in charge. A Safe Boss is one who does not abuse that role, one who shares power with the child in their care in every instance where it makes sense to do so. However, when a child gets to say "no!" in response to a direct instruction from a parent, this is usually dysregulating. Children intuitively know that they do not have the life experience, wisdom, and power to be in charge, so when they are given inappropriate power in a family system, their neuroception of safety is disrupted: It is scary for children to be in charge, to be bigger than the parent. A parent who is functioning as a Safe Boss knows how to set limits safely while also sharing power.

A few years ago, I worked with a dyad in which the adopted child, Polly, was having screaming meltdowns at least once a day. At these times, Polly would throw things at her mother and sometimes hit her. Mom would try to placate her, and when all else failed, she would lock herself in a closet, so as not to get hurt until Polly calmed down. She would, in essence, leave Polly when Polly was in her most intense distress and need of her mother. Her mother removed herself when her child needed for her to bring herself closer.

Figure 3.2 is the play creation constructed by Polly to represent her relationship with her mother. Notice that the symbols chosen for each are babies. Polly was adopted at 5. When she was performing well, her mother was totally available to her. When she became disrespectful, her mother became childlike herself. Part of the work for this family was helping the parent grow in her holding capacity so that her child would begin to see her as a Safe Boss, as opposed to a peer with a commensurate level of emotional maturity. As I got to know this dyad, it became clear that Mom was very comfortable being a secure base for her daughter. She would come into session and celebrate her daughter's perfect score on a math test, mastery of a new piece on the piano, or her ability to pull all of her hair back into a ponytail by herself. Independence was easily celebrated by Mom. Where Mom got stuck was in seeing her daughter's defiance as a cry for more help in her distress.

Often when I am unpacking the need-meeting roles of parents, it becomes clear to them which tasks around the circle come more easily for them and which might be more difficult. An amalgam of our own experiences—which includes but isn't limited to the ways in which we were parented, our education, our temperament, our personalities, and the way in which any traumas we have experienced have been encoded—can affect our ability to be bigger, stronger, wiser, or kind as

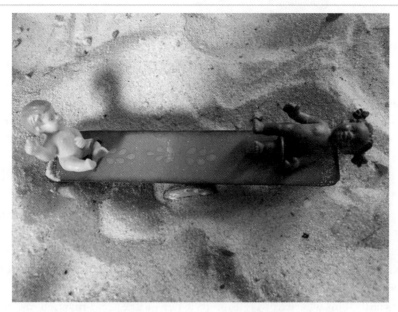

FIGURE 3.2. Who Is the Boss? Equals on the Seesaw.

we support our children's independence or their neediness. In fact, it is likely, to be expected even, that each of us is more comfortable on either the top of the circle (supporting exploration) or the bottom of the circle (welcoming our children back in their distress), making the other task more difficult for us. How do we grow an ability to hold the pain of the children in our care? The good news is that once we have acknowledged our own predisposition, we can intentionally cultivate responsivity to the other needs of the children in our care. In some cases, helping foster or adoptive parents to understand their own attachment history can be the key to creating a paradigm shift (Siegel & Hartzell, 2013). Uta is one such mother.

Uta is an adoptive mom who presented as kind and quiet during our meeting and expressed extreme doubt in her ability to be "bigger" than her adopted son, who often flew into rages in the home. She responded to his disrespect either with meekness or with intense anger, but always with a sense of helplessness that she could do anything to effect change. I asked if she would be willing to explore her own attachment history with me. We first spent time together developing a timeline. She had been raised by her grandmother in another country from ages 2 to 9, came to America for a brief period with her grandmother, and then joined her mother, who had married and moved to another country, when she was 10 years old. When I asked what she remembered about the first 2 years of her life, she was unable to give any kind of narrative about those years. The paucity of information itself was saddening for both of us and intensely disturbing to her, once she realized how little she really knew about her first 2 years. She began to reflect on how little coherence of her early life had ever been made. Uta started to understand that no Storykeeper existed for her during this time. When I asked her one of the first questions from a clinical adaptation of the Adult Attachment Interview (AAI), she again responded with a scarcity of information.

The question asks the interviewee to list five adjectives to describe the relationship between the client and their mother during early childhood (quantified as ages 5–12). Uta was unsure how to respond and asked if I wanted her to answer for the time she spent with her grandmother (ages 5–9) or the time she spent with Mom (9–11). We decided she should do both, over time. We started with the 2 years that Uta spent with Mom. Her first descriptor for their relationship was "polite." Uta went on to explain that there was never any yelling or anger between her and her mom, and that she herself was very well behaved. Uta then said "easy."

After Uta offered up the five descriptors of her relationship with her mother, the next question asked for an example or supporting story for each of the descriptors given. So I asked, "Can you give me an example of a time it was 'easy' between you?" Uta paused for a long while and then said, "Nothing really stands out . . . in fact, I should say 'blank' instead of 'easy.'"

Eventually, Uta was able to tell me that her mother had married and started a new life in a foreign country. Trying to explain the sudden appearance of a daughter after years without one would be awkward, so Mom asked Uta to pretend that her mother was her aunt. Reflecting on this experience with me, she was able to begin questioning whether or not her mother had actually been an attachment figure. Uta saw the Circle of Security, which we had explored together in a psychoeducational way, in a whole new light. She saw clearly how her mother supported her exploration, providing praise and encouragement when her daughter was able to "do for herself" or achieve in any way, but could not remember any significant moments of Mom supporting her in her neediness or distress.

I asked if there were times when she had felt afraid and Mom helped. "There was a skylift that went over the town where we lived. I remember a time that we went to ride the skylift. I was 9. It was Mom, my stepfather, and me. Each lift could only carry two people and my mom was afraid to ride by herself, so she went with my dad and I rode by myself." Uta was taught that she needed to be strong and independent all the time. Think again about the two basic ways that children get their needs met in their primary attachment relationships: support for their exploration (as they move out from us to explore the environment) and welcoming them back in their distress. Uta was not allowed to express distress. Does this mean that she did not have any? When asked directly if she could remember times when she had been scared, sad, or in distress, she was able to pinpoint one time when she had a nightmare and was allowed to sleep on the floor of her mother's bedroom. Beyond that, she stated, "Everything went along smoothly. . . . I just remember it being calm . . . well, blank." Using the language of Circle of Security, because it made "us" (Uta and her mother) uncomfortable for the child to be needy and dependent, she learned to mask her need.

In the worst-case scenarios, we can even become disgusted with our own neediness as a way to keep it quashed. This can help us to remain close to caregivers who can't handle our neediness. Growing reflective capacity in caregivers through instruments like the AAI is part of our clinical work and can encourage parents to grow self-compassion in the safe, listening, holding presence of the other and eventually earn a secure attachment. As Uta reflected, at times reexperiencing or potentially fully experiencing (for the first time) the pain of not having been fully accepted as a child, those reflections and feelings were held. She was able to take a step back from her unconscious dance with her son and decide which parts of her mother's mothering she wanted to perpetuate. Equally as important was Uta's growing capacity to acknowledge the patterns that she wants to change. Her mom's message to her was some version of *I should not have to hold your big feelings. I am unable to do so and it would be unfair of you to ask me.* Uta, now all grown up and with adopted children of her own, realized that she was communicating this same message when her children exhibited big behaviors or shared big feelings. After this important session, Mom went home to help her kids do their homework. It is a profound truth that as the parent makes new room within themself, the child takes new risks. Or, perhaps takes risks that had never been understood as such before. During out-loud reading time with her son, as he was reading about a female athlete, he stopped abruptly, looked up at his mom, and asked, "Is she as strong as you, mama?" Uta heard this differently than she had before. Instead of hearing it as a challenge, she heard it as a request: "Please be this strong for me, mama. The world is scary and I need an anchor." She sent me a picture of the page they had been reading. As she made sense of her own attachment history, she was hearing the needs of her children, for her to be bigger, stronger, wiser, and kind (a Circle of Security mantra), differently than she ever had before. As she develops compassion for her own neediness and experiences her own sadness about not having those needs met, she expands her ability to have compassion with her own children in their neediness, and to hold their experiences of sadness, anger, disappointment, and to make repairs when there are ruptures.

The handout entitled "Safe Boss Creed" (see Figure 3.3) can be printed out and used in sessions as a jumping off point for enhancement of specific parenting capacities or strengthening of practical skills sets. For example, if a parent feels that he is not able to set clear limits, he would benefit from conceptualizing this as one of the roles of a Safe Boss, and specific parenting procedures around limit setting can follow. The Creed can be hung on the refrigerator for the parent to read, reference, or rehearse whenever he needs to breathe in his role more deeply. There are some families in which big brothers or sisters, who may sometimes function as babysitters, begin to absorb some of these roles with those more vulnerable than themselves within the family.

Some parents I work with print out the Creed and review it in their quiet times, almost as a spiritual practice. Safe Bosses know what the people in their care are capable of and how to encourage them at their growing edges. Put another way, Safe Bosses know where to set the bar for those on their team. It grieves me to see a teacher, parent, or counselor pushing a child to do something that she is truly

THE SAFE BOSS CREED

Safe Bosses function both in authority and under authority.

Safe Bosses delight in those they lead.

Safe Bosses assign good intentions to those they lead.

Safe Bosses set clear limits when needed.

Safe Bosses share power when possible.

Safe Bosses use their power to protect those they lead.

Safe Bosses can hold all the big feelings of those they lead.

Safe Bosses can hold the hard stories of those they lead.

Safe Bosses provide instruction when needed.

Safe Bosses help those under their authority to practice new skills.

Safe Bosses earn the right to speak into the lives of those they lead.

Safe Bosses see the giftings in those they lead and know how to call them out.

Safe Bosses give the people they lead a clearly defined path for communicating problems, distress, or confusion.

Safe Bosses know what the people in their care are capable of and how to encourage them at their growing edges.

FIGURE 3.3. The Safe Boss Creed.

unable to do at this point in her development. The implied judgment that the child "should" be able to do this creates toxicity in the relationship. I see this early on when children have just come home from hard places. I work with many families who adopt children out of institutional settings. When a child has spent the first 10 years of life in an orphanage in which lying had been a necessary survival skill, parents often have compassion for this habit at first, but before long begin to feel bewildered, frustrated, or even disgusted. They will ask with frustration why their child is still lying when they have been in their safe, loving home, where rules and values are clearly stated and expectations are clearly set, for "a long time now." I often get this question when a child has been in an adoptive home somewhere between 9 months and 1 year. There are no researched guidelines for how long it takes children to develop a trust foundation after they have had a control foundation, but I'm pretty sure that 1 year of alternative experience . . . one-tenth of a 10-year-old's previous experience . . . is not long enough. Moreover, the question of what "alternative experience" means needs further unpacking. For hurt children to risk change, to risk trying out new behaviors, they must feel safe. And safety includes a lack of judgment. When a caregiver's "shoulds" do not take into account the child's origins or how the child has negotiated survival, the child does not feel understood and more than likely does not experience the neuroception of safety. This "mostly safe but" feeling impedes the child's ability to try out new behaviors.

Lying seems to be a behavior that is particularly challenging for parents in this regard. Parents will sometimes explain that the punishment for lying in their family will always be worse than the punishment for whatever a child is lying about. This may work decently well in a family where the child is securely attached, but with traumatized children this distinction only further arms the fear-based brain. The lying is a knee-jerk behavior, a habituated response that is wired into their neurophysiological reactions to stress. I am remembering a young man, Toni, who was brought home to a wealthy family in middle Tennessee after spending 10 years in an orphanage. The family had several younger children and were hopeful that he would function in a big brother role to the others. He would sometimes hoard food and he often told lies, even about things that didn't "really matter" according to the parents, or about things that were clearly untrue. The parents would ask, "Did you wash your hands?" after he went to the bathroom, and he would give an automatic response of "yes" even though the water had clearly not been turned on. They were bewildered about why he kept lying.

Eventually, my relationship with Toni had developed to the point where he felt safe and supported enough to share some of his experiences in the orphanage. I explained that I see lots of kids who lie and that there are usually some pretty good reasons why they do so. The lying helped them in certain ways in their old environments. I asked Toni if he could draw a picture of one way in which lying benefited him in the orphanage. He drew hands on a piece of paper and then slashed across them with red marker. When I asked him to tell me about his picture, he said, "In the orphanage, if you were caught being out of your bed at night, or fighting, you got lashings on your hands with a branch." (Toni was still learning English, and we came to understand that he meant a switch or sapling.) He explained, "You got 10 lashes if you were out of bed and 20 for stealing." I asked what his largest lashing had been; he said, "Fifty . . . my hands were bleeding." Sometimes he lied to avoid lashings, and other times it benefited him to take the blame for something he didn't do (another form of lying) to earn his way into the good graces of a peer who had access to resources he didn't. His adoptive parents knew nothing of these experiences in the orphanage.

I offered to help him share these pieces of his experiences with Mom, and as he did, I watched new understanding dawn on his mom's face. She moved quickly from a place of intense reaction when he lied to being able to say, "I know that you are still learning to trust that we are safe for you. When I ask a question, I'm going to understand that your first answer might not be the truth. But the door is open for you to come back as soon or as late as you realize the lie and feel safe to tell me the truth. I will thank you for telling me the truth and honor how hard it was for you to do so." Wow. The whole culture of their home began to change.

Soothing: The Journey from Other to Self

We know that for the young child, in particular, attachment figures are hugely involved in helping children develop right brain regulation as caring adults are meant to anchor and support the developing child in every way (Bowlby, 1969, 1973, 1980, 1988). Put another way, being able to soothe the self comes directly from first being soothed by "the other." There is general agreement in the field now that the attachment relationship provides the pivotal anchor for a child's development of affect regulation (Applegate & Shapiro, 2005; Hughes & Baylin, 2012; Fonagy, Gergely, Jurist, & Target, 2002; Schore & Schore, 2008). Whenever a caregiver can provide consistent repetitions of grounded, calming attuned responses when a child is upset, the more predictably the caregiver soothes, and the more secure the developing attachment relationship, which maximizes healthy hierarchical brain development (Cicchetti, Rogosch, & Toth, 2006; Fosha, 2003; Hatigan et al., 2012; Siegel, 2020).

Babies come out of the womb wholly unable to soothe themselves: They rely on the Safe Bosses around them to meet their needs. Fascinatingly, the visual focal point for a newborn is about 8–10 inches from their face. How far is that? It's about the crook-of-the-arm. When a baby boy is nestled into his caregiver's arms, in close, nurturing contact, baby and caregiver can open and close circles of communication that help both the mom and baby know and be known by one another. The baby begins to rely on feedback from his mother to provide interest and fun, to soothe and regulate. Play is a primary form of attachment behavior. Play is the glue that holds together a secure attachment relationship between parent and child (Kestly, 2015).

Babies come out of the womb wired for connection. From the moment the baby is put into his mother's arms, and the baby goes, "Ah, gah goo gah," and Mom goes, "Ah, gah, gah, goo, yah!"—right then the baby learns that he can impact the world, that he has a voice, and that he matters. Schore and Schore (2008, p. 14) talk about "right-to-right brain prosodic communication" as a powerful tool in increasing caregiver–child attunement and ultimately the child's regulation. Parents meet basic needs thousands of times in the first few years of life. The baby is hungry and Mommy feeds her; the baby is wet and Daddy changes her. Each of these moments of discomfort is met with soothing by a Safe Boss. However, what seems to make the difference between nurturing, adventurous, empathic adults and those who are more anxious or withdrawn is the quality of interactions that parents have during these moments of need meeting.

Some caregivers provide what we call "instrumental care"—they change the diaper in a "get her done" kind of way—while other parents take advantage of this arguably unpleasant task to play peekaboo, to tickle the baby's tummy, or to pick "toe berries" and pretend to eat them. The baby squeals in delight, which rewards the parent and encourages the parent to play some more. This symbiotic enjoyment wires the baby's brain more and more toward relationship and toward the expectation that relationship with others will be pleasurable, while rewarding Mom with her own competency surges around being able to soothe and delight her baby. This cycle creates neurochemical cascades of good feelings within and between parent and child. So, long before babies have words, they can know that they are delightful. We can show them their preciousness through play. Babies who get thousands of repetitions of need meeting learn to anticipate soothing. Each of my children developed in this way. When they were infants, they would wake from a nap in full-blown alarm mode, wailing at the top of their lungs. I would go bounding up the stairs as quick as my legs would carry me to pick them up, rock them, and soothe them, and tell them I was there and had them. They would take big, gulping breaths as they came back to regulation through closeness and eventually let out a sigh, communicating that they were settled. Around the 6-month mark with each of my three children, they would wake from a nap and begin to cry, but when they heard my footsteps on the stairs, they would stop . . . anticipating that the soothing was coming.

Anticipatory soothing is just as real as anticipatory anxiety. In fact, anticipatory soothing (in part encoded in object permanence) can mitigate a child's distress when facing something scary. The internalized working model of the parent *as* available even when they are not present can produce a powerful soothing response within a child who has received good enough parenting. The regulatory dance that happens with caregivers and their babies helps develop the baby's brain in ways that soothe and regulate the brain stem, providing limbic resonance and connection for the limbic brain, leaving the neocortex free to be cognitively curious about the world. Soothed, connected infants have an almost eerie ability to focus. When they are fed, snuggled, and grounded, babies can stare at their mothers or at other sights and sounds in the world with a stillness and a focus that allow for valuable learning about the surrounding world.

When I am helping caregivers make the paradigm shift from being managers of behavior to being co-regulators of their children, I will often show a series of three images of myself with my daughter when she was around 2. We had just gotten out of the car to go into Mammoth Cave when she bonked herself in the mouth with her sippy cup (see Figures 3.4, 3.5, and 3.6).

This was physically painful and emotionally upsetting to my daughter, so I picked her up and held her close, providing the prosody that helps to calm, paired with physical contact, and she began to regulate. She then put her hand on my collarbone and her thumb in her mouth and continued to anchor her physical body to mine as she soothed herself using just as much of me as she needed. I nursed

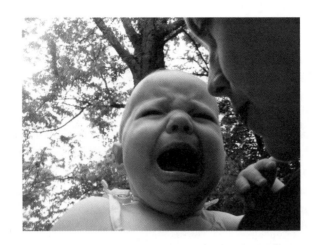

FIGURE 3.4. Dysregulated.

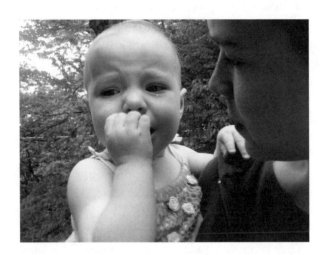

FIGURE 3.5. Connecting.

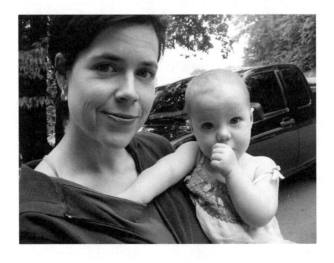

FIGURE 3.6. Co-Regulating.

Madison for the first year of her life, and while she was nursing, she would put her hand on my collarbone. After I weaned her, when she was upset, she would put her hand on my collarbone and suck her thumb. Six months after that, she no longer needed to put her hand on my collarbone; she just sucked her thumb to soothe; and 6 months after that, she no longer sucked her thumb. She had internalized an ability to soothe herself, *but her self-soothing came only after thousands of repetitions of being soothed by the other.* This process continues over the lifespan with lengthening time spans during which children are able to regulate themselves. Having said that, there never comes a time when we operate completely independent from the need to be soothed by an other. I still call my mom when I am outside of my window of tolerance for stress. Children who have had thousands of repetitions of being soothed by the other in early childhood return to their optimal arousal zone more quickly in adulthood than adults who did not get these neural pathways laid down as children.

When children have not had a "good enough" caregiving system, when they have not experienced the thousands of repetitions of nurturing care that extend our window of tolerance for stress and help teach us how to regulate our distress, they simply do not have the neuro-scaffolding to soothe themselves. This is why adoptive parents can have 10-year-olds in their home who may be able to make perfect grades on their math tests when they are limbicly calm, but who respond with infantile regression and disorganization when somatically or socially emotionally upset. These children did not receive the co-regulation of an *other* earlier on, so have no internalized soothing to draw on. The importance of early attachment figures in helping children learn affect regulation cannot be overstated. I work with many families who have the joyful experience of receiving their adopted child into their arms right at birth. In some cases, they even get to cut the cord. These parents can have the hardest time making paradigm shifts as they see difficulties begin to arise in their children. They can get mired in feelings of parental shame or guilt, preoccupied with questions of whether or not they have caused their child's dysregulation through their own "bad" parenting. Since I have found that this focus impedes their ability to shift, I begin to offer parents whatever information I can surrounding the *in utero* injuries that their baby may have undergone. I will sometimes refer parents to *The Secret Life of the Unborn Child* (Verny & Kelly, 1988), which is an excellent read and makes the argument strongly for how lifelong regulation patterns, among other things, are strongly influenced by the *in utero* experience.

I paint the picture for parents of a fetus growing in the womb of a mother who is eagerly awaiting the birth of her baby. The first full-body vibrations that the fetus absorbs are the regulating rhythms of the mother's heartbeat: thump, thump . . . thump, thump. Over time, the baby's heartbeat moves to mirror the mother's heartbeat, coming into synchrony. If the mother is hiding the pregnancy and therefore not maintaining the nutritional input that will be healthy for the baby, or if the mother is in a domestic violence relationship, her heartbeat may be unpredictable, sometimes steady and sometimes racing, with potentially massive releases of cortisol flooding into the baby's bloodstream. Mom's neurochemicals are bathing the baby's brain. Six months into the pregnancy, Mom and baby come into neurochemical alignment. If Mom struggles with depression and anxiety and has lower serotonin and dopamine levels herself, this neurobiology may be mirrored in the baby. At the very least, the same absence of health-giving neurochemicals may be reinforcing an environment of deficiency for the baby's developing brain. This early neurobiological insufficiency can translate into a core somatic re-experiencing pattern of lack. The core belief that can develop out of this *in utero* experience is "there will never be enough for me." This belief, somatically encoded, can contribute to patterns of self-sabotage in relationships later in life. For some, no matter how much love or nurture is given, the individual still believes it is not enough or may be removed at any moment.

A plethora of research has brought us to a new understanding of the importance of the prenatal period in shaping the central nervous system across the lifespan. This discussion surrounding the critical period for the release of prenatal hormones that set the baby up for emotional and physiological stress regulation later in life also primes the mother's brain for the challenges of attuned caregiving (Glynn & Sandman, 2011). All of this information suggests that providing support and intervention for pregnant mothers may need to be the earliest focus of our interventions.

Loss of Voice

One of the most critical experiences for a neglected or maltreated child can be the titration of intimacy and trust-building with a Safe Boss. Well cared for babies also know the power of their own voice. When they experience discomfort, they communicate their distress about being hungry, cold, wet, or lonely by crying and someone comes. They cry and someone helps . . . pretty powerful stuff. We call this crying "aversive cuing," as it brings us to the baby, in part, because we want the crying to stop, we want the unpleasant experience to end, and our often immediate response does the trick in teaching infants the power of their voice. But what happens if the baby cries and no one feeds him, or is wet and no one changes him. What does this baby learn? That no one will come, that his voice doesn't matter, that crying makes no difference.

A groundbreaking study for its time, Infants in Institutions (Provence & Lipton, 1962) followed a group of 75 institutionalized infants and a group of 75 infants raised in families and performed multiple forms of assessment. They found that, overwhelmingly, the babies who were raised with an absence of maternal care experienced adverse effects. One significant finding was that when a baby cries for 30–60 days consistently within an institutional setting, they lose their voice—they simply stop crying.

The idea of eventually giving up is reinforced by Ed Tronick's work, particularly what has come to be called the Still Face Experiments (Montirosso, Cozzi, Tronick, & Borgatti, 2012). In these experiments, the researchers focused one camera on the mother's face and one camera on the child's face, and they encouraged Mom to play with the baby. It is difficult not to smile as you watch the beginning of one of these clips, as the mom and child are usually in a sweet dance of cooing, giggling, verbalizing, and delighting in each other. Then the researchers ask the mom to blunt her affect, to wipe any expression from her face, to give the baby a blank stare. At first the baby is confused and seems to be thinking, "Maybe you didn't hear me, or maybe you were distracted." Sometimes I suspect the baby is saying, "I know you think I am the most delightful thing ever—you must be distracted. Let me show all my cuteness, let me try again" and she makes another squeal. The baby first tries harder. If Mom remains unresponsive, seemingly disconnected from the baby's cues, the baby gives up. She becomes disorganized. She may begin to drool, may lose coordination of her limbs, may begin to cry or stare at the wall. She becomes disorganized without the organizing presence of her other. This research has powerful implications for the importance of attuned, responsive caregiving.

Children who do not have their neediness supported begin to tune out from their own distress. The body's signals that we have a need deserve a place of honor . . . they deserve our attention. So, if my stomach gurgles because I am hungry, I try to listen to my body's cue and am even grateful to my body for letting me know what it needs. However, paying attention to a need when the need is not being met sickens the soul and exacerbates pain. Children who are hungry and remain hungry learn ways to disconnect their minds from their bodies. They begin to see need, and certainly expressed need, as a weakness. Once children believe that expressed need is a weakness, they have very few options left for how to get their needs met. They must do the job themselves. These children learn that they must control everything because they can't trust others to meet their needs and keep them safe. This control can be externalized and manifested as a need to control others, or it can be ruthlessly applied internally. The child may decide to control every expression of difficult emotion through sublimation, pretending the feeling doesn't exist, morphing it into something less vulnerable, or compartmentalizing it. We can be very creative in learning to mask our needs when they aren't getting met. This context helps us understand how habits of sneaking or hoarding food, lying, and stealing can become not just reasonable choices for such children, but the safest choice. In essence, the masking of needs (mainly done unconsciously) embodies a profound way of giving up on the relationship with a Safe Boss. Children who have a Safe Boss develop a *trust* foundation (Erikson, 1993). They believe that the world can be trusted and that caregivers will be responsive. Children who have not experienced a Safe Boss develop a *control* foundation. I see many, many children with this foundation. Their core belief seems to be, *I must control everything at all costs, or I'll die*. Once we understand that control feels to the hurt child absolutely vital to his survival, we can better understand why he is always demanding a third option even when a couple of options he normally likes have already been offered. This can look like the parent saying, "You have two choices: You can wear the red shirt or the blue shirt" and the child screaming, "I want the purple shirt." It really isn't about the purple shirt; it's about the lack of trust in the Safe Boss relationship. Safe Boss status with foster and adopted children must be earned, and it takes time—tons and tons of time.

Safe Boss as Reinforcer of the Child's Goodness

Many years ago, I created an activity called the Good At . . . Game (Goodyear-Brown, 2002). At the time, I was working in an inner-city school, and the intervention invited a child to create a bowl-shaped container to represent himself. He then filled the bowl with gems and was invited to take the gems out of the "self," one by one, while identifying out loud one thing he was good at.

I have been providing support for a 6-year-old boy, Jimmy, who carries a great deal of anxiety all the time. If he has a negative thought about a friend, he thinks he is bad and spirals into hurting himself. He generally can only identify feelings of happiness in relation to those in his life, as he believes that any other big feelings, such as frustration, sadness, or anger, are bad feelings and mean that he is a bad boy. He has trouble being kind and compassionate with himself, although he works hard to be this way with others. He relies heavily on his adoptive mother as both a secure base and a safe haven, and I understood that asking him to focus any energy on articulating his own positive attributes would be challenging and perhaps create anxiety for him, so I invited Mom to join us. Mom was delighted to do so and helped Jimmy make his container after she had made hers. She got him a large ball of Play-Doh, and he said, "I just want a small one." They worked together to make one that was small. He then chose one large stone and said, "That's all that will fit." While using concrete materials and speaking matter-of-factly about the amount of space available for positive affirmations, his negotiation with the play materials paralleled his constant negotiation with himself around his internal struggle with seeing his own goodness.

Mom and I played the game first, taking turns saying things we were good at for each of our stones, allowing him to observe and get used to the idea of the game. He was able to verbalize, "I am a good friend" for his stone, but he immediately jumped down from the table, ran over to the tray of golden nuggets on the other side of the room, and began sifting his hands through the nuggets. Mom and I joined him in the nugget tray, understanding that this play brought regulation and a necessary break for Jimmy. After a few minutes of playing with something else in the room, Mom asked if he wanted to play Good At again. I invited him to change the game in any way he liked. His face lit up and he said, "I know!" He came back to the table and took his Play-Doh person bowl and his mother's Play-Doh person bowl and stuck them together. Then he made a hole in the wall of Mom's bowl and worked with great concentration to make sure that it was big enough to let the gems through (see Figure 3.7).

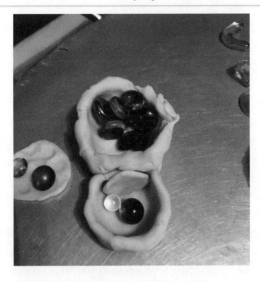

FIGURE 3.7. Sticking Together to Explore Self.

It was, for me, a beautiful example of Jimmy's need for more support from his Storykeeper, his secure base, to be able to explore positive things about himself. Mom would talk about a positive quality in herself that she also saw in Jimmy and then put it in her bowl and let it roll through into his. He was unsure of his "I am's" and asking for more of Mom's shared experience. Instead of saying, "You are a kindhearted boy," she said, "We are good at being kind to our friends." She became his conduit toward more self-compassion, while remaining the holder of his story. Sticking together with Mom in this way mitigated his approach to the scary content, which for him was self-affirmation.

Safe Boss as Holder of the Hard Story

Traumatic stress disorders are rooted in anxiety. In the case of children who have been adopted, there can often be a core anxiety related to worth: the guiding, pounding question that is too terrifying to ask out loud for fear of the answer is "Am I worthy of belonging?" Many of these children feel thrown away and wonder if this means that they are garbage. One of the hallmarks of posttraumatic stress is an avoidance of people, places, and things. In play therapy, the playroom becomes the microcosm in which the child wrestles with the avoidance, giving us the unique opportunity to work with the avoidance by putting "skin on it" through the symbols in play and working with the symbols over the course of play therapy. Traumatized children can identify with certain symbols that remind them of their vulnerabilities—these we sometimes refer to as "self-objects" (Goodyear-Brown, 2010). The symbol itself can become both an anchor for activation within the child and then a mitigator for the child's approach to whatever is psychically upsetting to him or her about the symbol. Many examples of inviting parents into the story-keeping process are shared in my book *Trauma and Play Therapy* (Goodyear-Brown, 2019). More strategies for enhancing the storykeeping role of parents will be given in Chapter 9.

When we are exploring Safe Boss behavior with parents, the Hoberman Spheres can be a powerful metaphor for the relationship between parents and children, offering a visual for concepts like containment and being able to hold big feelings. It was, of course, a child who showed me the power of the metaphor to illustrate this relationship. At Nurture House, we have a larger Hoberman Sphere and a smaller one. The larger sphere is big enough for a 4-year-old to get inside when it is fully expanded (see Figure 3.8).

Jillian was a 7-year-old girl who had grown up in a household where Mom was chronically ill. Sometimes her mother was present and available, and other times Mom had to stay in the bed because of a flare-up of her autoimmune disease. Mom acknowledged the potentially insecure attachment caused by her inconsistent availability and brought her daughter for play therapy to help the mother process the effects of her chronic illness on her daughter. During our second session, Jillian noticed the spheres (Figure 3.8). She took the larger of the two and expanded it. Here is the transcript of the conversation that followed:

PARIS: You made it big!

JILLIAN: Yep, it's as big as it can get.

PARIS: It can't get any bigger.

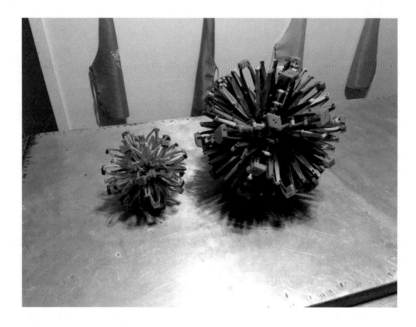

FIGURE 3.8. Mom–Child Hoberman Sphere.

(*Jillian goes over to the basket that holds the smaller sphere, pulls it out, and then inserts it inside the fully expanded, larger sphere.*)

PARIS: You put the little one inside the big one.

JILLIAN: Yeah, there was room for it to go in.

PARIS: I wonder if it's safe inside the big one?

JILLIAN: Look! (*Takes the bigger sphere and compresses it until it is small enough to surround the small sphere so tightly that you can't even see the small sphere anymore.*) This is safe!

PARIS: Oh, the little one feels safest when the big one is snuggled up really close all around.

JILLIAN: Yeah . . . but sometimes (*she fully extends the big sphere again*) this one can roll right out. (*She works hard to make the big sphere remain expanded on the floor and then she flicks the small one, also resting inside the larger one, and has it roll out and away from the larger sphere.*)

PARIS: Oh, the little one rolled away. . . .

JILLIAN: Yeah, it might be awhile before the big one goes to find it.

[Jillian went on this way, creating various play scenarios. In some of them, the "bigger, stronger, wiser, kind" sphere held and protected the little one. In others, the little sphere slipped right through and was alone. The constant changing of bigness and smallness in this young girl's play left me with a visceral impression of a relational yo-yo. Eventually, I began to wonder out loud about the patterns I was seeing.]

PARIS: I'm noticing that the big one is sometimes tucked right around the little one and other times the little one can roll right through, Wonder what the little one likes best?

JILLIAN: (*talking on a high-pitched voice—speaking as the little sphere*) Be bigger than me! But not too big!

Soon after this session, I had a parenting session with Mom and she explained that when her pain is at its worst, she becomes really big: speaking very sharply to Jillian and overreacting to small annoyances. I was able to describe Jillian's play pattern, but halfway through my description, I said, "You know, I'd rather show you. Would you like to see the spheres? She was eager to do so, and as soon as I had put the small sphere inside the big one and compressed the larger one to be close around the little one, she began to cry and said, "I want to be able to hold her close this way." We then talked about practical ways to help Jillian still feel held when Mom is in her worst moments of pain. Mom returned for a parent consult several weeks later and talked about how important the visual image of compressing to become a *bigger but not too big container for her daughter* had been. We cannot overestimate the importance of visual imagery for parents as well as for children.

Internalizing Safe Boss

Safe Bosses find ways to make their presence felt, enhancing the attachment across time and space, even when they are not together with the people they lead. In a trauma and family context, children who have been neglected or maltreated may have a very blurry schema of the internalized parent. Sometimes this manifests as separation anxiety or an ambivalent attachment in which the parent becomes confused by the "come here, go away" pattern as the child's neediness and quick anger cycle. I often describe the ambivalently attached child as desperately needing the parent while being desperately angry with the parent, and unable to fully articulate either state of being.

In other systems, children will not have successfully navigated Piaget's object permanence task. "Llama Red Pajama" was one of my children's favorite bedtime stories (Dewdney, 2015). Mama Llama's explanation to little llama sums up object permanence beautifully, "Don't you know I'm always near even if I'm not right here." In both of these cases, children can benefit from having transitional objects (Winnicott, 1953) that concretize the relationship between parent and child when they need to be separated due to the school day, or because of a parent's work outside the home or even out of town.

Transitional objects can be especially important for children of divorce, who go back and forth between two homes regularly. Often in TraumaPlay when we are working through the goal of Soothing the Physiology, we will further enhance the role of parent as partner through the use of transitional objects (Goodyear-Brown & Andersen, 2018). These objects can provide anchors for the felt safety of physically absent parents, offering concrete connection to the feelings of nurture and soothing that the child may experience when in the physical presence of a parent. Figure 3.9 is an example of Love Connectors. My son taught me this intervention

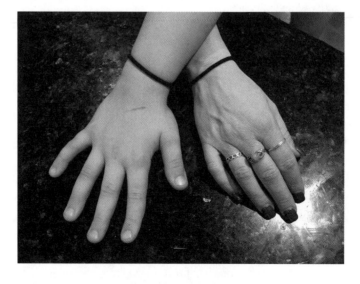

FIGURE 3.9. Love Connectors.

several years ago. I was packing to go on one of my 36-hour round trip speaking trips. As Nicholas, my preschooler at the time, watched me pack, he spontaneously said, "We need more love connectors!" Not knowing exactly what he meant but understanding that this was the expression of an underlying need, I reflected, "We *do* need more love connectors. Shall we go find some?" He took my hand, scooted down off the couch, and led me all around the house, until we were standing in front of my jar of ponytail holders. He exclaimed, "There they are!" He opened the jar, pulled out two matching ponytail holders, put one on my wrist and one on his wrist, and seemed satisfied. The next morning I was dropping him off at preschool and we were holding hands on the way in. Our love connectors (ponytail holders) were touching and he said, "Our love connectors are powering up!" While I was gone, we FaceTimed a couple of times. Each time he asked me to hold my love connector up to the screen and we powered them up. As I edit this manuscript, we are in the midst of the global pandemic that has forced many of us, as therapists, to move to virtual work. I have never been more grateful for this intervention, as I am often supporting parents and children in creating love connectors through the screen, or having both the child and myself create connectors that maintain the strength of our relationship virtually as we are physically separated. Another way to do this intervention would be to ask parents to have beads and string (or, if doing telehealth, dried macaroni or cheerios, anything that can be strung). In the session, a child and parent can take turns finding two beads of the same color and adding one to each necklace as they verbalize one positive quality they share. For example, Mom and child might both have beautiful brown eyes, and this shared beauty could be celebrated on both necklaces. Both parties can then wear their necklaces during those times when the child is visiting the other parent's house.

There are also times when a child has developed separation anxiety connected to a trauma. A child who was previously largely independent may begin to cling to their primary parent. In these cases, it benefits the system to incorporate the playful practice of small distances between parent and child. There is a sweet book called *Pouch* (Stein, 2009) that we use as the foundation for a parent–child exercise at Nurture House. The book is about a mommy and a joey. After we read the book, we place the child right next to the parent, perhaps even held in the mother or father's arms, and pretend the child is Joey in the pouch. Then we roll a large wooden die and however many dots are on the die, the child takes that many hops away from the parent. Together, we all then experience how safe or unsafe that distance feels to both the parent and child.

Celebrating Positive Growth in Safe Bosses and Their Families

I recently worked with a family that was in great distress at the time they came to Nurture House. Their son Adam was so dysregulated that multiple sessions had to happen in the car before he was stable enough to even enter Nurture House. When I met the family, Adam had been asked to leave his specialized school, was having difficulty leaving the house, was unable to regulate for longer than an hour or two, and had responded in complex and problematic ways to the multitude of psychotropic medications that had been tried. We baby-stepped our way for months into establishing safety and security. This first required a balance of helping Adam feel that his parents and I delighted in him, while also protecting him from his own tendency to lash out and hurt others when he became dysregulated. This baby-stepping entailed helping the parents set and hold some new clear limits with Adam. They also became very skilled at celebrating his vulnerability whenever he would share a feeling, and understanding how hard some of the new behavior patterns were for him.

After we got to the place where this young man had almost extinguished his violent behavior, was experiencing some sense of competency and mastery, and had enrolled in a new school program that was helping him to feel socially connected again, I asked the family to create a sand tray to show their journey thus far in treatment. The sand tray is often a very safe space for families, as it has clear boundaries, allows for joint attention to a task (as opposed to intimate relational exchange), and encourages right brain hemispheric communication (Carey, 1999; Homeyer & Sweeney, 2016). It was important that they be able to reflect on how much movement had been made and how hard each family member had worked to change. We also wanted to refocus on the goals for ongoing work.

In one corner of the tray, Mom and Dad created the image shown in Figure 3.10. Mom described feeling helpless and desperate as she watched her child regress into infantlike behaviors. She and Dad are the figures on their knees, and Dad's

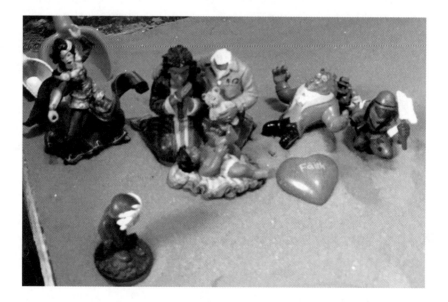

FIGURE 3.10. Waving the White Flag.

head is missing (this is a ceramic figure and unfortunately it has been dropped). The client is represented by the baby on his back in front of them. Mom also placed a beast in the tray and talked about how devolved their whole family situation felt when they began therapy. Mom talked about her choice of the heart as a nod toward her belief that your heart starts to live outside your body whenever you have children, and how hurt her heart was feeling as she experienced an inability to stop her son's pain. On the far right is a soldier kneeling down waving a white flag. Mom talked about a sense of giving up and crying out for help when things were at their worst. I wondered out loud about there being no shelter for the family, and Mom agreed, "Yes, it was as if we were in the middle of a desert, at the mercy of the elements." I asked if she could title this part of the sand tray, and she called it "Beasts Waving the White Flag" (see Figure 3.10).

In the middle of the sand tray, Mom had placed a cheerleader and a rescue helicopter (see Figure 3.11), both representing the role of the therapist (me) in their journey. I was glad she saw my interactions with the family in this way, as both encourager and helper. In terms of parallel process dynamics, as I offered encouragement and help when Mom and Dad were dysregulated and overwhelmed, they began to encourage and help their son in new ways. I really see our role as therapist as putting our arms around those who put their arms around the child. If the two main tasks of Safe Bosses—supporting children's exploration and welcoming them back in their distress—are to be internalized by parents, it helps tremendously for them to be modeled by the therapist. When parents are feeling confident and equipped to try out something new in their parenting, we support their exploration. When they

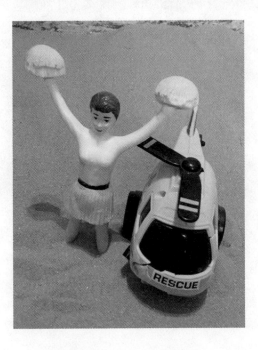

FIGURE 3.11. Safe Boss Roles.

return, we celebrate their risks and results or hold their distress. The many repetitions of these interactions with parents equip them to provide these kinds of support for their children and believe that these parents have expanded their abilities to do more and more of these things as their son or daughter needs them.

In the other corner of the tray, I asked Mom to show me the family as she perceives it currently. At first, Mom chose a healthy, typical-looking "cool kid," the African American figure standing and smiling to the left of the doorway to their home. The sister is represented by the little girl with the soccer ball, and Mom spoke about how her daughter was getting to spend more time in age-appropriate activities now that their family had a healthier daily rhythm (see Figure 3.12). Mom chose Wonder Woman to represent herself and Batman to represent Dad, and talked about the feelings of strength—even superhuman strength—that she and her husband have used together to pull them through this tough time. She also chose the Superman figure and talked about how the whole family has performed superhuman feats to get them to where they are right now. And where are they? When I asked Mom to title this part of the tray like she would title a book, she decided to call it, "Back in the World." She recognized that there is still a long way to go until they will be ready to fly on their own, but there was such hope in her tray: hope that each member of the family had the internal resources needed to continue moving forward.

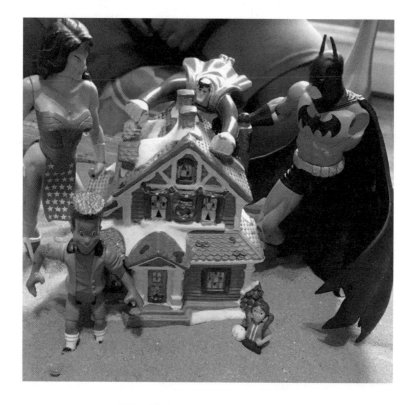

FIGURE 3.12. Back in the World.

Safe Boss as Parallel Process

Clinicians can model all of the Safe Boss behaviors for the families in their care. The Cascade of Care begins as the therapist delights in the parents equally with the children, sets clear limits, shares power, assigns good intentions, provides clear pathways for communication about problems and feedback, and the like. The therapist models the dimensions of healthy leadership that can become part of the family system's way of relating. We, as therapists, may represent different aspects of the Safe Boss at different points in treatment. We are sometimes cheerleaders, sometimes holders of the story, sometimes offerers of a different perspective, sometimes limit setters.

Figure 3.13, a photograph taken at Camp Nurture, shows one of our young campers at a time when her body let us know she needed to rest. One of her buddies offered a pillow and her lap for this little girl to rest on. The second buddy for this child got behind the holder and began to braid her partner's hair, providing nurture to the one providing nurture to the child. It wasn't until long after Camp Nurture was over that I found this photograph. I find it a beautiful representation of the parallel process dynamics and the Cascade of Care we've been exploring. When we as therapists hold the holder, the traumatized child is also held.

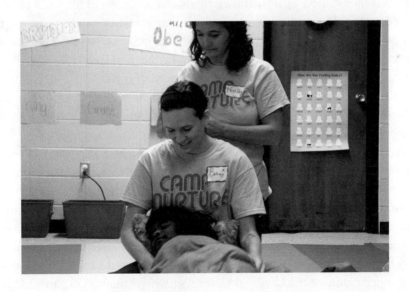

FIGURE 3.13. Holding the Holder.

CHAPTER 4

Helping Parents Understand Themselves to Understand Their Children

If there is anything that we wish to change in the child, we should first examine it and see whether it is not something that could better be changed in ourselves.
—C. G. JUNG, *The Integration of the Personality* (1939)

Parents are people, too. In fact, they were people long before they became parents. The whole amalgam of their experiences, right up to the moment that they bring their child to therapy, represents a lifetime of navigating the intersection of nature and nurture. Nature includes the parents' genetic makeup, their temperament, their level of introversion/extraversion, their primary love languages, and their physical health. Nurture includes the parents' whole set of caregiving experiences, their relational circles of communication with their own mom and dad early in life and currently the nurture that they do or do not receive from their romantic partners or co-parents, their priorities based on Abraham Maslow's Hierarchy of Needs, and the unique dimensions of whatever academic and relational education they have absorbed.

Helping parents make connections between their own earliest attachment relationships and those they have with their children now is a powerful but complex piece of the work. Parents can be offered tools that encourage integration of early experiences through both left and right brain ways of knowing. Using symbols, sand, clay, or art during the reflective process aids in the integration. Some therapists believe that the line between treatment with children and treatment with their parents is clearly demarcated. I disagree. I think the line is quite blurry and should be. I think the continuum of treatment with the minor child requires us to shift parents' paradigms, practice new skills sets, and grow their containment abilities, as they will ultimately be the holder of their child's hard story. This will require them to be able to touch their own pain in order to hold their child's pain. We generally refer parents for individual treatment when there is intrapsychic work to be done or deep trauma processing work for the parent. We do this, in part, so that the child is not further overwhelmed by a parent's big feelings during conjoint work. However, when the trauma that a parent may be processing in their own therapy is one shared by the child, and especially when the psychological or behavioral fall-out of the trauma is the reason for the child's referral to treatment, a coherent and shared narrative of events will become part of the healing work for both the child and the therapist. To this end, expanding the parents' reflective capacity is helpful and requires making connections about the ways that they were parented, the ways of relating to their own children that arose from such parenting, and what patterns they want to change or get rid of altogether. This may involve processing some trauma content with you, the child therapist.

This work is not for the faint of heart. It requires vulnerability and courage to look at our own early attachment relationships and the confusion, hurt, terror, anger, or sadness that may mark them. To this end, we call this "RAW work for parents." RAW is an acronym for Reflective Attachment Work and offers an expansion of the verbal processing done in question-and-answer assessments of adult attachment, by inviting right brain involvement through the use of sand tray miniatures and expressive arts. This cross-hemispheric, externalized processing serves two purposes. The first purpose is to expand parents' access to all the ways of knowing that are available to them by using the whole brain (Badenoch, 2008; Badenoch & Kestly, 2015; Homeyer & Sweeney, 2011). The second purpose is to begin inviting them to experience the power of the symbolic, metaphor-based work that will be woven in and out of their child's treatment process.

Child clinicians need a solid grounding in attachment theory in order to understand how to intervene in the family system. Mary Ainsworth's Strange Situation experiments (Ainsworth & Bell, 1970; van Rosmalen, van der Veer, & van der Horst, 2015; Main & Cassidy, 1988; Main, Hesse, & Kaplan, 2005) were foundational to our understanding of attachment patterns. She put together a series of experiences that were meant to stress the child and activate the attachment system, and then observed how the child and parent coped with the stress. If we understand that a child's attachment behavior is a strategy for staying close to the parent for survival, a biological imperative, then we begin to make sense of the patterns that emerged from her work. The experiment included eight situations. The parent and child would enter an unknown room, and the researchers would observe how the parent and child navigate their introduction to this new space; eventually, a stranger would enter the room and the researchers would watch whether or not the child checks in with their parent for reassurance that the stranger is safe, if and how the child interacts with the stranger, and so on. The crescendo of the experiment occurs when the parent departs from the room, leaving the child with the stranger. In time, the parent reenters the space, and the researchers observe the behavior of the child at reunion. Careful attention is paid to the child's behavior during separation from and reunion with the parent.

What has emerged is a set of attachment styles that have proven consistent across cultures. I have a very simplified way of describing these to parents, and every time I do so, I watch the wheels begin to turn. Parents are often reflecting on their family of origin attachment dynamics before reflecting on their current nuclear family dynamics. When the child with a secure attachment to his parent comes into the room and is connected with the parent, the two explore the space together. The securely attached child normally references the parent when the stranger enters, and may interact with the stranger if the parent gives cues that this is safe to do. The child may have some distress at the parent's leaving, but is easily soothed and/or redirected by the stranger. When the parent reenters the room, the child runs to the parent, eager to be picked up, and reconnects easily, often showing the parent something he had been doing while the parent was gone. The child with an ambivalent attachment is likely to cling to her parent, not wanting the parent to leave the room, and remain in distress for most of the time the parent is gone. When the parent returns, the ambivalently attached child may run directly to the parent and demand to be picked up, but once picked up, push or hit the parent. This "come here, go away" pattern of behavior is a hallmark of ambivalent attachment; the avoidant attachment pattern is the most difficult for me to watch. In this dynamic, the parent and child enter the room together, but the child is likely to play independently and the parent and child may be experienced as disconnected from each other. When the parent leaves the room, the child keeps playing—giving no outward sign that he cares the parent is going. When the parent returns, the child continues to play, offering no indication that he cares the parent has returned. But if you put a heart rate monitor on that child, his heart rate is going wild at the moments of separation and reunion. He has just learned to mask his neediness from his parent, because it is not the best strategy for staying close to that parent. The child may have experienced rejection when needy in the past, either by this same parent or, in foster or adoptive situations, by a birth parent. This dynamic is incredibly difficult with adopted children who are placed in a family in which the parent is more comfortable with supporting the child's independence than in welcoming the child in her neediness. Adopted children with an avoidant attachment style are miscuing their parents that they don't need them, and most adoptive parents want to be respectful of a child's need for independence and therefore may not foster some reversion to earlier dependency needs, either out of confusion surrounding the child's cues or because it is simply easier to support her current independent behavior. Finally, a disorganized attachment style is one in which the changeability or volatility of the parent has been so great—the parent is abusive, is in active addiction, or is dealing with a serious mental health issue—the child isn't able to come up with a strategy that consistently works for staying close to the caregiver.

Five and Dive: Cross-Hemispheric Reflection

A powerful reflective exercise for helping adults reflect on their own childhoods is the Adult Attachment Interview (AAI). The AAI was created by Mary Main and is a series of 20 questions aimed at helping an adult reflect on their early attachment relationships (George, Kaplan, & Main, 1985, 1996). One such question asks the parent to give five descriptors (adjectives) of his relationship with his mother in early childhood (the period of time between ages 5 and 12). When I ask this question of parents, I give them a blank piece of paper and the space and time to make a list. Many parents report that the first two or three descriptors come easily and then there is a pause. Paying attention to the pauses can help us circle back with curiosity later. Once the parent has written down all five descriptors, I ask that he share the list out loud. Then I offer a circular sand tray and sand tray miniatures, and ask the parent to choose a symbol to represent each of the descriptive words. Our extrapolation of this question about the parent's relationship with his primary caregiver in early childhood is called the "Five and Dive." This simple activity expands the parent's ways of knowing and the expression of his early experience from being mainly centered in the logical, linguistic, linear, "just the facts ma'am" left hemisphere of the brain to embrace right brain ways of knowing. I prefer to use a circular tray for this work, as each aspect of the parent's attachment relationship with his parent was probably experienced on a cyclical basis. Using a circular sand tray also inhibits the tendency we have to put things in order, to make them more hierarchical, or to arrange the miniatures in order by the frequency of certain kinds of interaction. We know that volatility does not need to be expressed as frequently as nurturing care for it to become equally embedded in our patterns of navigating the world and staying safe. Sometimes parents develop a new awareness of their own parents' patterned interactions with them as we process the circular sand tray. If you do not have a circular sand tray, a paper plate filled with sand can work.

In fact, paper plates filled with sand serve nicely in a training setting. It is an expected aspect of our training program to have new clinicians engage in a process of reflection regarding the attachment dynamics within their families of origin. TraumaPlay therapists embrace parallel process work. Therapists who work at Nurture House have experienced the interventions themselves that we ask them to guide parents through. One reason for this is that we are then able to resonate deeply with the difficulty of exploring one's own stuff. I recently had a very talented and compassionate therapist who works at a children's advocacy center and helps the most vulnerable children and their foster and adoptive parents to heal from trauma come through TraumaPlay training. At the end of the advanced weekend, she left me a little card that said, "Thank you for helping me work on my $%@#." Other TraumaPlay therapists have joked that we should perhaps hand out T-shirts that say, "TraumaPlay: Where you work on your $%@#," because we spend time in training looking at our own attachment histories, our own triggers, and how we refill our own compassion wells when they run low. Supervisors in the TraumaPlay model hold individual stories of the clinician's early attachment relationships, both with their families of origin and their nuclear families now, so that the clinician can learn to hold the stories of the parents' attachment relationships within their family of origin and guide them into an interactional shift with their children. A therapist's work on their own person is valued at Nurture House and often provides the kind of corrective emotional experiences we hope clinicians in training will be able to offer to the families in their care as they hold their client families' stories. Moreover, clinicians are given time and space to reflect on their own earliest attachment relationships and to experience the different qualities of learning that occur when we reflect using left brain, linear, linguistic processes and when we reflect using right brain symbolic, iconic, and somatic ways of knowing. Figure 4.1 shows the Five and Dive sand tray of one of my clinicians.

The five adjectives listed were *absent, confused, nurturing, fun,* and *adventurous.* She chose the following symbols to represent each adjective: For *absent,* she chose a soldier. For *confused,* she drew a question mark in the middle of a piece of paper and placed this at the center of the tray. For *nurturing,* she chose a swan with babies protected on its back. For *fun,* she chose a playful young boy who looks like he should be climbing a tree. For *adventurous,* she chose E.T., the endearing extra-terrestrial, in a bike basket (see Figure 4.1). She explained that he was often deployed and physically absent. She also offered a story related to the blended family dynamic as support for the confusion she felt. Notice that a couple of her adjectives referenced more challenging dynamics of the early relationship (*absent, confused*), while some of the others are qualities all children hope to have in their relationship with a

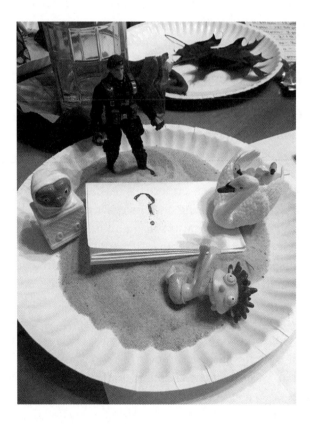

FIGURE 4.1. Confusion and Protection.

parent (*nurturing, fun*). This balance of the positive and negative aspects of the relationship is one of the hallmarks of a grown-up who has earned a secure attachment in adulthood, whether or not she had one in childhood. As we listen to the choices of adjectives given by the clinician and the example story that supports each one, a pattern begins to emerge. These patterns tell us about the early attachment relationship that the person in our care (clinician or parent) experienced. This can be tremendously important for treatment, as understanding the attachment patterns experienced by the parent in early childhood colors all of that person's current interactions with the child in her care.

An overabundance of either positive or negative attributions assigned to the early attachment relationship is usually an indicator that the grown child remains stuck in some way. When all five descriptors are glowingly positive, the difficult aspects of the parent's early relationship may still be too difficult to look at. The grown child may continue to have an allegiance to a parent, a concern that she will be disrespecting that parent if she says anything negative about the parent, or some other defense mechanism that makes it impossible for her to look at hard things from her family of origin. When all five descriptors are completely vilifying, this also tells us that the grown child has unresolved issues and may not feel fully individuated or out from under the parent's control yet.

I worked with a dad who taught me a lot about how entrenched we can be, even as adults, in the stories that we were told about our caregiving or the stories we learned to tell ourselves to survive. Matt, a father seeking help because he felt unable to connect to his two elementary-school-aged daughters, completed the Five and Dive sand tray. His adjectives for his relationship with his mother in early childhood were *warm, nice, fun, kind,* and *loving.* I asked him to give me an example of a loving moment in his relationship with his mother. There was a long, long pause. He seemed to be searching his memory and finally said, "Well, there was a time when we were in a grocery store parking lot. I was about to run out in front of a car and she pulled me out of the way." If this was the most loving moment Matt could remember, the statement pointed to his need to believe all positive things about his childhood at this point in his development. It was rewarding to walk alongside Matt as he began allowing himself to acknowledge hard things about his own childhood. His mother worked constantly, and he was often lonely. As he began to allow himself to feel some of the pain he experienced at her absence, he was able to become more present for his own children.

Window of Tolerance Cross-Hemispheric Work for Parents

Most mental health professionals are familiar with the Window of Tolerance (Siegel, 2020; Ogden, Minton, & Pain, 2006). The concept has become a cornerstone in understanding individual reactions to stress. While this content is especially important when dealing with traumatized and attachment-disturbed families, it is useful for all parents. The exploration, in the case of parent–child communications, is the interaction of the arousal responses of the parent and the regulation of the child, and the arousal responses of the child and how these reactions affect the parent.

While this thought might be daunting to parents, it is important to acknowledge that children are continually neurocepting something. In a perfect world, children would be neurocepting nurture all the time from their caregivers. All people, and therefore all parents, move into and out of various states of regulation daily. While we may strive to remain within our optimal arousal window, daily challenges can kick us up into hyperarousal, down into hypoarousal, or even into a state of collapse. The attachment dance requires children to feel their parents neurophysiologically so that they can employ the most effective strategy for staying close to them at all times. If a mom is in a state of hyperarousal, the neurocepting offspring may become quiet and more obedient, or over time, may move toward hyperarousal of their own. The neuroception of safety is most effectively absorbed from parents who are regulated in their own right. Helping parents learn about and reflect on their own Windows of Tolerance for stress, as well as how they tend to operate when they are outside of their optimal window, can lead to important paradigm shifts in the way parents see their own stress and the stress of their children. As a play therapist, I also deeply value the knowledge and understanding that come from cross-hemispheric work, so our approach at Nurture House to psychoeducation around the Window of Tolerance uses both words and symbols to access information from both the left and right hemispheres of the brain. Figure 4.4, which appears later in the chapter, is a script we use to help lead parents through an exploration of their own Window of Tolerance dynamics. The parent's Window of Tolerance work provides a scaffolding for parallel process work with children and teens within the home. Three separate reflective exercises are discussed in this section: WOT Are You Doing?, WOT Are You?, and Create Your Ideal Window.

The handout labeled "WOT Are You Doing?" outlines the kinds of parenting behaviors we are likely to see when parents are in their optimal arousal zone (we call this our "best parenting self"), when they are in a state of hyperarousal (and are overresponding to the situation), and when they are in a state of hypoarousal (and are underresponding to the situation). The therapist can print out the handout (see Figure 4.2), have parents circle the behaviors that sound most like their responses, and join the parents in their curiosity about which way they tend to swing: over-responding or underresponding, how they feel about the pattern that emerges, and co-create the beginnings of a plan for how to move back into their optimal arousal zone from a state of either hyper- or hypoarousal more quickly when they find themselves kicked out of it. They then frame their initial psychoeducation around Window of Tolerance concepts and their parenting behaviors.

It is again parallel process work: As parents recognize their own patterns and work to shift them, they develop deeper compassion for the difficulty that the attempt to change presents, for themselves and then for their children. I have identified patterns in my own life that I have wanted to change, and when I respond

WOT ARE YOU DOING?

OVERRESPONDING	BEST PARENTING SELF	UNDERRESPONDING
HYPERAROUSAL	OPTIMAL AROUSAL ZONE	HYPOAROUSAL
YELLING	REGULATING MY EMOTIONS	WITHHOLDING ATTENTION
BARKING OUT ORDERS		WITHHOLDING AFFECTION
SLAMMING DOORS	GIVING CLEAR POSITIVE INSTRUCTIONS	SLEEPING A LOT
STOMPING AROUND		CHECKING OUT
SPEAKING CRITICALLY	SETTING CLEAR KIND LIMITS	GIVING UP RULE ENFORCEMENT
CONTROLLING MY KIDS	ASKING FOR WHAT I NEED	
HOVERING		SIGHING A LOT
RUSHING AROUND	LISTENING WITH COMPASSION	FEELING FUZZY & UNSURE ABOUT HOW TO RESPOND

This exercise helps you reflect on your Window of Tolerance for stress
and how you tend to react when you are kicked out of your optimal arousal zone.
Circle the behaviors you engage in most often.
What does this say about how you respond to parenting stress?

FIGURE 4.2. WOT Are You Doing? Worksheet.

again in a manner that is not the way I wanted to respond, it reactivates my compassion for how much harder it must be for children to change. As we extend compassion to parents in the process of change, meeting them just where they are, the corrective emotional experience that this represents for them positively influences their ability to extend compassion when their children fail.

The second exercise is meant to help parents explore, cross-hemispherically, their own Window of Tolerance for stress. We call this tool "WOT Are You?" (see Figure 4.3). This worksheet can be printed out as a template for the exercise, or the parent can simply fold a piece of paper into thirds, as she would fold a letter to

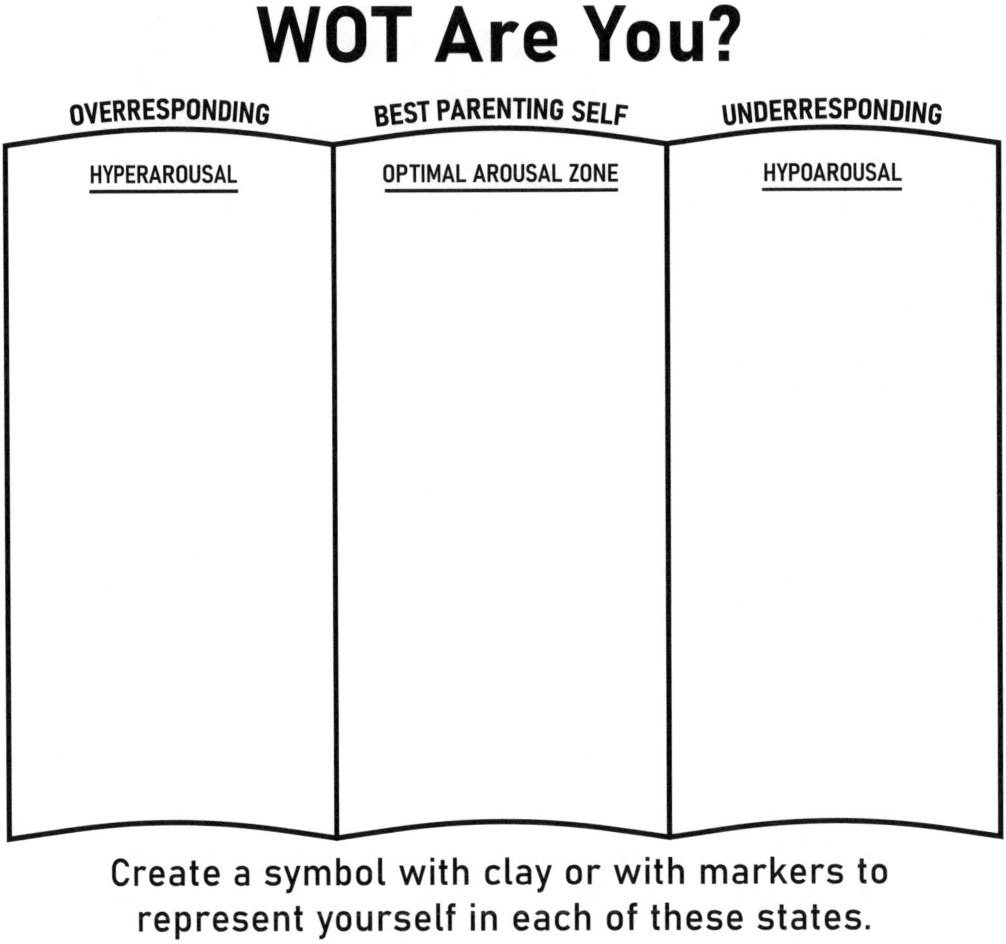

WOT Are You?

OVERRESPONDING	BEST PARENTING SELF	UNDERRESPONDING
HYPERAROUSAL	OPTIMAL AROUSAL ZONE	HYPOAROUSAL

Create a symbol with clay or with markers to represent yourself in each of these states.

FIGURE 4.3. WOT Are You? Cross-Hemispheric Work.

put it in an envelope. In the left-hand panel of the trifold paper, invite the parent to create a symbol for herself when she is in hyperarousal. In the middle panel, invite the parent to create a symbol for herself in her optimal arousal window. In the right-hand panel of the trifold, invite the parent to create a symbol for herself in hypoarousal. The Window of Tolerance script (see Figure 4.4) is also available to therapists to help guide the activity. This exercise can be done in a variety of ways or with several iterations. In the first exercise, the parent may be prompted to create or choose symbols for the way they experience themselves within various arousal states. In a second pass at the same concepts, the parent may be prompted to create or choose symbols for the way they believe their child, the whole group of

Window of Tolerance Script

This exercise is meant to encourage cross-hemispheric reflection on the caregiver's hyperarousal, hypoarousal, and optimal arousal states. Offer the parent the WOT Are You? handout or a piece of paper that may be folded into thirds, like a letter. Also have markers, clay, and Play-Doh available. Say the following:

Being a parent is hard work. You have already identified some behaviors you engage in when you are your best parenting self, and patterns of over- or underresponding when you are kicked out of your Window of Tolerance.

In the middle panel, draw or create a symbol to represent you as your best self. This usually involves feeling grounded, connected, and able to give and receive healthy communication while creating, responding, and functioning well.

In the left-hand panel, create a symbol to represent yourself when you move into hyperarousal. Hyperarousal usually involves over-reactivity. Some parents report having shorter tempers, feeling like they are running on a hamster wheel but not getting anything accomplished, or are too stressed to think when they move into hyperarousal.

Create a symbol in the right-hand panel to show me what you are like when you move into hypoarousal. Some people describe sluggishness, procrastination, and withdrawal.

Remain present with curiosity and quiet attention while the caregiver completes this portion of the work. Then invite the parent to talk about their symbols and why they were chosen. After processing the three symbols, state the following:

The goal is for us, as caregivers, to be able to realize when we are outside our optimal arousal window (the place where we feel like our best selves) and to get back into it as quickly as we can. The next exercise will help you hone in on what you need to stay within this window more often.

FIGURE 4.4. Window of Tolerance Script.

children who live in the home, or their parenting partner, experiences the parent in each state of arousal. This work often leads to rich reflective attachment work, developing the parent's capacity to take the perspective of other family members who must navigate their arousal states while becoming more attuned to becoming more skilled at accurately identifying the parent's own movement into and out of these same states.

Once the parents have worked through their sense of self when they are experiencing each state of arousal, they often are motivated to explore how to remain, more often, in their optimal arousal zone. Each of us has a unique combination of experiences, rhythms, and relationships that keep us within our Window of Tolerance. To this end, we explore what a parent needs, in the rhythms of her work life, her home life, and her self-care, in order to remain grounded in the parenting role as frequently as possible. The directions are as follows: "We are going to create a personalized window that shows what you need to stay within your Window of Tolerance. Your window may be one pane of glass or have many panes; it may have a frame made of wood or metal. It may need curtains, blinds, or a pull-down shade to provide extra protection or boundaries. Use the questions below to reflect on what you need to stay within your Window of Tolerance. Then create a window that shows the things you need to be your best parent self."

I have created a window for my work life (see Figure 4.5) and one for my home life (see Figure 4.6). Each of these shows the balance of activities that keep me grounded. Family time is an enormous anchor for me, as you can see from the window I made for family.

These are simply meant to serve as examples. Offering parents this exercise helps them articulate what self-care looks like in practical terms, and can serve to highlight what may be missing altogether. Individual windows can be made for individual areas of life: family, work, friendship, community involvement, hobbies, etc.

You may need to support parents in looking honestly at how their current rhythms of life compare to what they see as optimal. Remind them that it is difficult to know where you are headed if you don't have a vision or a goal. The windows are simply one way to cast vision.

It is also worth talking to parents about setting goals to achieve more balance and margin so that some progress can be made in that direction. Some parents won't have a template for what balance or nourishing rhythms of life look like. My optimal arousal zone for work would have me seeing no more than 15 clients a week (I see way more than that now), doing several supervision sessions a week (I do way more than that now), allotting protected time for note writing, reviewing records for those times when I have to provide court testimony, and so forth and 4 hours of creative time per week—which feels like a pipe dream right now. But knowing what I'm going for has helped me say "no" to additional clients and set boundaries around some creative time each week. We've all got to start somewhere. The "What Do You Need to Stay within Your Window of Tolerance?" (see Figure 4.7) can help parents in this process. After parents have filled it out, you can print out the blank

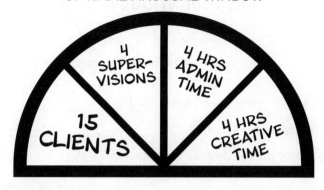

WORK WEEK
OPTIMAL AROUSAL WINDOW

4 SUPER-VISIONS

4 HRS ADMIN TIME

15 CLIENTS

4 HRS CREATIVE TIME

FIGURE 4.5. Created Window of Tolerance: Work-Related.

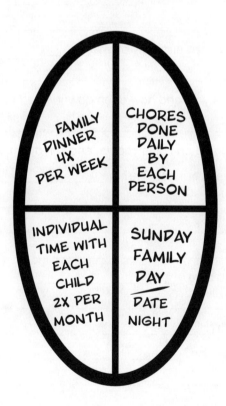

FAMILY
OPTIMAL AROUSAL ZONE

FAMILY DINNER 4X PER WEEK

CHORES DONE DAILY BY EACH PERSON

INDIVIDUAL TIME WITH EACH CHILD 2X PER MONTH

SUNDAY FAMILY DAY
DATE NIGHT

FIGURE 4.6. Created Window of Tolerance: Family-Related.

What Do You Need
to Stay within Your Window of Tolerance?

How many hours of work, per day, are optimal for you? _____

If you work by appointment, how many appointments per day are best for your work/life balance? _____

How much administrative time do you allot for yourself? _____

How many hours of sleep do you need? _____

Which people in your life do you need to see regularly? _____

_____

What rhythm of quality time spent together is optimal for you to have with a romantic partner? _____

With each of your children? _____

_____

What kind of time? What kind of rhythm? _____

_____

What sort of foods do you need and how often? _____

_____

What sort of exercise helps you, and how often do you need it? _____

_____

How much time do you spend on social media, and is it optimal? _____

How do you unplug or check out from life? _____

_____

What do you do for fun? _____

_____

What do you consider self-care? _____

_____

How regularly do you do it? _____

How do you leave work behind? _____

_____

FIGURE 4.7. What Do You Need?

windows template labeled "What Do You Need to Stay in Your Optimal Arousal Window?" (see Figure 4.8). This exercise is meant to function in a parallel process way as well, where clinicians have explored these concepts for themselves, help parents to explore them, and then help the parents help their children to explore them. To this end, creative clinicians can make the whole activity more playful by offering pizza boxes, pieces of fabric, cardstock, pipe cleaners, craft sticks, and clear plastic wrap or other see-through material to be the window panes and window frames. This can be, in some cases, a rich activity for the family to do together in a session.

Threat Level Assessment

Another part of the reflective process for parents as partners in child therapy involves helping parents better understand their own levels of perceived threat. I travel a good deal to speak. As part of that, I am often confronted in airports with screens displaying the current threat level of terrorist attack. The airports in the United States use a 5-point, color-coded system for communicating how dangerous it is to fly at any given time. It is called the Homeland Security Advisory System and maps threats in this way: The least scary code is LOW (green) and means that there is a low risk of terrorist attack. The second level is GUARDED (blue), which translates to "general risk." The yellow bar is labeled ELEVATED and stands for "significant risk"; then comes HIGH (orange) and the most alarming level is SEVERE (red). For several years after September 11, 2001, the airports stayed at threat level orange nearly all the time, increasing a traveler's wariness and weariness.

Our therapists talk about these threat levels and apply them to parenting. We keep the colors but replace the words with a 5-point scale. We have developed a blank version of this scale and use it frequently in both sessions and workshops with parents. We invite parents to reflect on their experiences and identify the problematic behaviors of their children along this continuum. What are the threats to your equilibrium or groundedness as a parent? What we perceive as threatening or alarming is unique to each of us. Disrespect is a general category. While many parents may see disrespect as a threat to their position or a sign that they are not in control, the form that disrespect takes can vary, as can the extremeness of response by a parent. One parent might see a teenager's rolled eyeballs as extreme disrespect. For this parent, the rolling eyeballs of his teen might set off a cascade of upset and consequences from the parent, making it a 5 on his threat-level scale (see Figure 4.9). Other parents can ignore rolled eyeballs—they might mean almost nothing to a parent, but if the teen doesn't check in through a text when she is going to be delayed, that may constitute a 5. The therapist guides the parent's reflection by saying, "Which of your children's behaviors are annoying to you . . . it would be a low-level annoyance. You don't like it, but you can easily live with it." Parents might respond with things like a son leaving his shoes in the living room or a daughter

What Do You Need to Stay in Your Optimal Arousal Window?

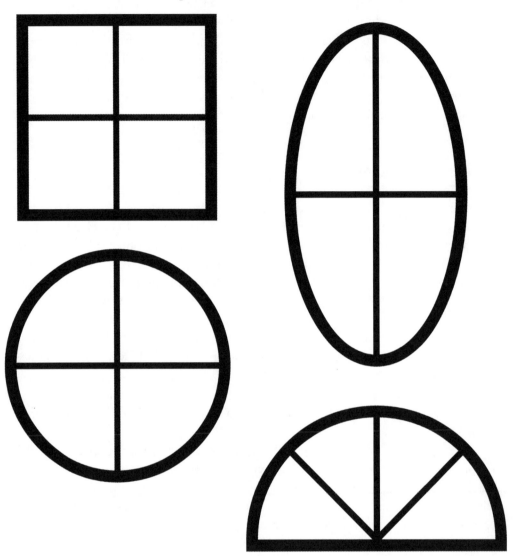

Choose a window to represent your family life. Fill in the panes with the time per week you want to spend engaged in various family activities. Feel free to use additional windows to do the same with other categories such as work life, romantic partnership, leisure time, social life, and nourishing personal practices. Feel free to add or remove additional panes as needed.

FIGURE 4.8. Optimal Arousal Window: Create Your Own.

Each parent has different behaviors that trigger them.
While some parents may see their teenager's eye rolling as a 1,
creating a low risk that they might lose their tempers quickly,
other parents may see eye rolling as a five and they might get
triggered really fast. **Write your child's difficult behaviors in the boxes
based on how triggering/ threatening they are to your sense of calm.**

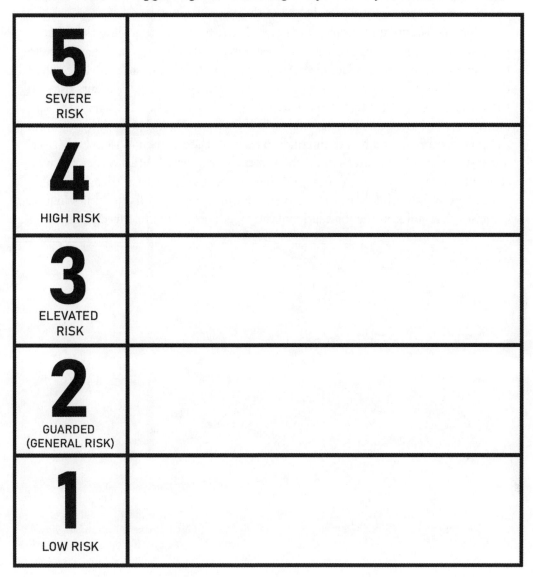

FIGURE 4.9. Parenting Threat Level Assessment.

clicking her tongue while doing homework at the kitchen table. The therapist then asks, "Can you identify a behavior that is more difficult for you to deal with? You can still maintain your cool, but you sort of have to remind yourself to stay cool." And the final prompt is "If you think about the moments when you've really lost your temper, said things you regret, or acted like a child yourself . . . what was going on? How would you describe the behavior that dysregulated you?"

Helping parents understand themselves is the first step in helping them better understand their relationships with and responses to their children. Staying true to the value we place on the Cascade of Care, TraumaPlay therapists experience all of these exercises in their own training process and then gently guide parents through these exercises in order to expand caregivers' self-awareness. This expanded self-awareness helps the parent better understand their own Window of Tolerance and to be a safer container when their children move outside of their Windows of Tolerance. As parents better understand the severity of perceived threat associated with some of the big behaviors of their children, it becomes easier for them to remain curious around the child's underlying needs. Future chapters will offer skill-building exercises that build on the foundational introspection offered in this chapter.

CHAPTER 5

Helping Parents SOOTHE

A DEEP DIVE INTO CO-REGULATION STRATEGIES

As clinicians grow, they are exposed to multiple theories of change and multiple models for helping families heal. Clinicians who treat traumatized children need skills sets for helping clients leach the emotional toxicity out of their trauma content. They also need skills for enhancing attachment relationships. Frequently, I have the conversation with clinicians about whether the child needs to be processing the traumatic events first or enhancing attachments first. Although there is no one answer to this question, and certainly the guiding question "What can the system hold?" is relevant here, in the TraumaPlay model we prioritize enhancing the role of parents as partners, with this needing to occur before processing trauma content whenever there is a willing adult. We view the current caregiver as the Storykeeper for the client, and we want to do everything we can to enhance the caregiver's ability to hold the story while collaterally building the child client's trust in the caregiver's ability to do exactly that. Another section of this text will dive into expanding the storykeeping capacity of caregivers; this chapter instead focuses on the role of parents as soothing partners, as co-regulators of the client's physiology. Many parents have trouble believing just how positively powerful they can be when they embrace their role as external modems, or co-organizers of their child's experiences.

SOOTHE is an acronym for a set of strategies that I began developing, in collaboration with Linda Ashford, from the International Adoption Clinic at Vanderbilt Children's Hospital, and Patti van Eys, who was then the director of the Center of Excellence for children in the State of Tennessee's custody. All three of us participated in a pilot project funded through Vanderbilt University in 2007. We had all worked with complex trauma systems and were interested in exploring best practices for children with significant externalizing behaviors who had experienced multiple caregiver disruptions. We had also all been trained in Parent–Child

Interaction Therapy (PCIT) through Cincinnati Children's Hospital and were familiar with a skills-driven, behaviorally oriented approach to working with this population. I myself was steeped in attachment-based interventions and wanted to see a significant focus on the parent as co-regulator. We debated whether or not our work should maintain a behavioral focus or an attachment focus, and after sitting in this discomfort through several meetings, we decided that the answer was "yes" . . . and "yes." We would rather equip parents with both sets of tools than to deny them either. So, we got to work designing the SOOTHE strategies (Goodyear-Brown, 2010). Then we entered into our second round of real discomfort as we tried to design a pathway, a rubric by which parents could answer this question: When do I use behavior management and when do I SOOTHE the child in my care? At last, I landed on a guiding question for caregivers to ask themselves when they arrive at the crossroads of behavior management and co-regulation: Is the child in his Choosing Mind?

In live training environments, I offer my daughter Madison (who is now 14) as an example. When she was 3 years old, she was delightful but also strong-willed and carried some anxiety that could cause dysregulation. Let's pretend that it is 9 o'clock in the morning on a Friday. Madison has had a good night's sleep and a healthy breakfast. She is regulated, and we are playing with puppets in our home's bonus room. It is time to leave the house, so I say, "Please put your shoes on, sweetie. It's time to go to the store—and then we'll go to the park." She may have no problem putting her shoes on immediately, but if she dawdles significantly, or says "no," or ignores me and keeps playing, I have to ask myself the question "Is she in her Choosing Mind?" I review the last 12 hours and say "yes." In terms of Maslow's hierarchy of needs, she has had all her basic needs met, is well rested, is connected with me and regulated, and has been cognitively engaged with me in storytelling with puppets as well. So, I am going to give her two choices. When I am tweaking this intervention for children with attachment issues or trauma history, I offer these two choices: "You can choose to put your shoes on by yourself, or I can help you to put your shoes on." The choice here is really between completing the behavior independently or choosing support from the caregiver in some way. This choice rubric can be especially important for foster and adopted children who are learning to trust that their caregiver will provide help when they need it. For my Madison, who has a secure attachment to me, I may instead say, "You have two choices: You can choose to put your shoes on quickly, or choose to take your time—if you choose to take your time, we won't have time to go to the park after the store." Either Madison will put her shoes on quickly, which will be good for both of us, or she won't and that will still be good learning for her because her thinking brain was online when she made the choice between the two options. The natural consequence of losing time at the park because she took so long to put on her shoes will still be good learning.

Let's contrast that with a scenario in which I am dealing with the same 3-year-old child, but now it is 9 o'clock at night, we have been running around all day, Madison didn't get a nap, neither one of us has eaten properly, and I'm exhausted, too. I say, "Madison, please put your pajamas on, it's time for bed." She dawdles, says "no," or ignores me. If I persist, "You have two choices. You can put your pajamas on quickly or you lose your book at bedtime," I am setting her up for failure. She has outlasted her ability to regulate herself, and she needs me to come in closer and co-regulate her more effectively. She has lost her capacity for conscious choice. In practical terms, this may require the parent to see the child as at least a couple of chronological years younger during times of stress than they would see the child normally. I am going to approach 3-year-old Madison, at 9 P.M., more like a 1-year-old than a preschooler. I'm going to hold her pajama bottoms open for her, and say, "I'm remembering about you that you did not get a nap today . . . it's been a long day. Mommy will help—you put one foot in . . . good job! Now put the other foot in . . . good job! Now let's snuggle." When children are not in their Choosing Mind, because they are tired, overwhelmed, underfed, undercuddled, or overstimulated, it is the parent's job to come closer and provide greater structure.

The SOOTHE strategies are a codification of the co-regulation skills that can become critical for parents to employ when their children are not in their Choosing Mind. I will unpack these in great detail below, as well as offer a couple of concrete tools for parents to use in application and practice, but first let's consider the expanded acronym:

S = Soft tone of voice and face
O = Organize
O = Offer choices and a way out
T = Touch and physical proximity
H = Hear the underlying anxiety
E = End and let go

I always like to start explaining these strategies by acknowledging that none of them require a knowledge of rocket science. Indeed, many of these skills are things we may employ frequently, but offering all of them in a conscious way when they are needed can be difficult, and the probability of being able to provide these co-regulation strategies in real time when a child is escalated is greatly improved through in-office practice with the therapist, followed by homework and bringing scenarios back to the therapist to troubleshoot together.

Soft Tone of Voice and Face

Soft tone of voice may seem like a no-brainer, but it can often require quite conscious intentionality. When a child raises his voice after being given a direction and says, "NO, I WON'T," if the parent matches that with a "YES, YOU WILL!," the parent will have matched the child's escalation and there is nowhere to go but upward. If, however, the parents can anchor below the child—this does not mean whispering (as a whisper tone is actually triggering for some of our clients with sexual abuse histories)—by grounding themselves, parents have the best chance of de-escalating the child. The idea of being an anchor for the child is a powerful one for some parents. It is important that we don't underestimate the importance of symbols and metaphor for parents as well as for children. I worked with a mom who had great trouble seeing herself as bigger, stronger, wiser, and kind. When her child began to escalate, she would feel adrift in self-doubt regarding how to intervene. She would first ask nicely for her child to calm down, and when the escalation continued, she would end up yelling. She had talked in circles with me around this pattern. One day, I invited her to create a sand tray to show the process of escalation between them. I then offered the idea of anchoring below the child and asked Mom to choose an anchor from the sand tray shelves. Once she found the symbol that resonated with her, she held it in her hands for several seconds. I asked her to hold it, to notice the shape of it with her fingers and the weight of it in her hand. Then she put the object in the sand tray. The next week, when she returned, she said, "I don't know what it was. Every time I felt like yelling this week, I would remember holding that anchor and feeling its weight. I kept saying to myself, 'Be the anchor.'" During the following session, she stated that she had continued to practice anchoring her daughter. She said, "I think I needed to see it, to absorb it visually, before it really sunk in." The fact that her portals for absorbing the head knowledge would include seeing the visual symbol and feeling its weight was surprising to her, and a good reminder to me to tie parent coaching to the learning style of the parent in front of me.

Neurolinguistics research has taught us that people learn in different ways. Some absorb information most easily through auditory learning (hearing), others through visual learning (seeing the concepts illustrated, having a clear line of sight to the speaker they are learning from, following along with written handouts, etc.), and still others need to be kinesthetically involved, physically experiencing the concepts being taught before they will feel fully equipped to implement them or regurgitate them for a test. My early writings highlighted the importance of targeting therapeutic interventions for children through all three learning portals, but it is equally important to pull in alternative forms of learning for parents as well. Expressive arts therapies offer multiple portals for helping parents absorb new information and make movement therapeutically. When parents are having a difficult time shifting their paradigm, moving from one therapeutic medium (talking) to another (writing, referencing pictorial representations of concepts, and creating symbolic representations of the treatment focus through art or in a sand tray) can allow for a powerful shift. Particularly in relation to sand tray work, parents can choose figures to represent a feeling, thought, or response pattern that seems problematic and then physically begin to move figures around, shifting the placement of one figure next to another, removing things completely from the tray, or incorporating additional symbols that change the feeling, thought, or response pattern. The three-dimensional shifting of icons in the sand can aid the internal paradigm shifts we are hoping to support within the parent.

Returning to the idea of anchoring below the child, I encourage parents to slow everything down—practically speaking, we practice having them spread their feet shoulder width apart, breath in deeply, slow down their cadence, and deepen their tone. The handout entitled "Anchor Below Your Child" (Figure 5.1) codifies these skills.

I often ask parents to imagine themselves as a mama gorilla at the zoo. Have you ever observed a mama gorilla? She has an amazing capacity to remain placid in the face of great chaos. The baby monkeys may be pulling on her, jumping on her back, scrambling around in rough house play with one another, but she just lies there—chewing on some vegetation. Nothing phases her . . . unless real danger arises. Then she can become fierce. Sometimes in my worst moments, when I most feel like losing it with a child in my care, I picture that mama gorilla, and it helps me to stay grounded.

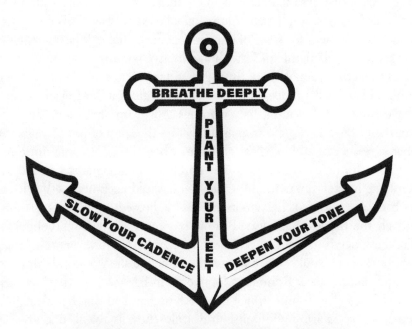

ANCHOR BELOW YOUR CHILD

FIGURE 5.1. Parent as Anchor.

Conscious control can be exerted more easily over the tone of our voice than over the tone of our face. The additional attention paid to soft tone of face in the SOOTHE strategies began when I was introduced to some pretty fascinating research by Seth Pollak (Fries & Pollak, 2004; Pollak, Cicchetti, Hornung, & Reed, 2000; Pollak & Sinha, 2002). He took photos of a woman making her most scared face and next her most angry face. Then he morphed these two images by tens of percentages inside a computer program and ended up with a continuum of faces that would include an image that was 90% angry and 10% scared, 70% scared and 30% angry. He then showed the whole series of images to a group of children with traumatized or anxious brains and a group of typically developing children, and over and over again, the children with traumatized brains would see the anger in the faces sooner than the children with more typical brains. This finding makes sense if we have a rich understanding of the hypervigilance symptoms that accompany trauma. The neurophysiological response of the brain to scary stuff is to encode the scary stuff and remain on the lookout for it, so it can be avoided in the future. Visual displays of anger may imply that even more scary stuff, like being yelled at, called names, or physically hurt, may be on its way. This constant scanning of the environment for signs of danger becomes a habit. The soft tone of face can be especially challenging for foster and adoptive parents.

Take Elizabeth, the mother of three grown biological children, as an example. Elizabeth and her husband decide to adopt a child from a hard place. They eventually have Ronnie, a 9-year-old boy who has grown up amid domestic violence, placed in their home. Over and over again, across the span of the 27 years that she raised her now successful biological children, when things became tense and she wanted to scream or overrespond to her children's behaviors, she would grit her teeth. Gritting her teeth was useful to her—she would keep her teeth gritted until she was back in control of her emotions, and it helped her to successfully regulate through the hardest moments. Ronnie has some challenging behaviors, and when Elizabeth needs to regulate, she clenches her teeth. However, in Ronnie's first home, his birth mom would clench her teeth just before she would call him a "selfish asshole" and slap his face. Ronnie's adoptive mom had no idea that her clenched teeth were a trigger for Ronnie. Once Elizabeth understood that her clenched teeth triggered a fear-based arming response in Ronnie, she was able to find another way to regulate. The tricky part of this work is that sometimes the clinician is simply joining with the parents in a process of being detectives together, trying to clarify what facial patterns may feed the fire of a child's upset.

Tone of face work requires some nuance and playfulness, and there are several ways clinicians approach this at Nurture House. One of our simplest interventions involves a handheld mirror and some dry erase markers. The mirror is one that I found at a yard sale. It has gold edging, and while one side offers a typical reflection, the other side magnifies the reflection. We have the parent hold the mirror far enough from his face that his whole face is reflected in the mirror. Then we offer the dry erase markers to the child and ask her to add anything needed to show the parent's most angry face. The child draws the elements on the mirror itself (a quick wipe of a paper towel erases the marker from the glass), and the parent's reflection usually ends up looking ridiculous. This allows the element of humor to mitigate a serious conversation about how parent and child react to one another (Franzini, 2001; Fox, 2016; Fry & Salameh, 1987; Garrick, 2005, 2014; Isen, 2003; Newman & Stone, 1996; Nezu, Nezu, & Blissett, 1988). Humor is a powerful way to decrease stress hormones (by increasing oxytocin release; Kirsch et al., 2005) and generally improves your mental and physical health (Berk, Felten, Tan, Bittman, & Westengard, 2001; Nasr, 2013; Overholser, 1992). Shared humor can connect people and help titrate the approach to hard things (Fritz, Russek, & Dillon, 2017; Hasan & Hasan, 2009; Gladding & Drake, 2016; Goldin et al., 2006; Wild, Rodden, Grodd, & Ruch, 2003). The most common addition to the parent's face in anger is a pair of angry eyebrows. We also keep stick-on eyebrows and mustaches at Nurture House, and these are often used during this part of the parent training in the SOOTHE strategies.

During one such conversation in our own home about what we communicate with our faces, my daughter, who was 6 at the time, said, "Mommy, I love your sparkly eyes . . . but sometimes they turn fiery, and I don't like your fiery eyes." Out of the mouths of babes comes the affectual impact that children experience based on the facial expressions of their parents. It is impossible to truly hide our somatic state from our children, who are wired to sense the current availability of their Safe Bosses. Mask work can also be done with parents alone or with parents and children together. One of my favorite prompts for mask work around soft tone of face goes as follows: "Design the outside of the mask the way you think your child perceives you when you are angry." Once the parent has completed this work, I offer the prompt "Design the inside of the mask to show all the feelings and thoughts that are swirling inside of you when you are making that face." Again, moving from a verbal exchange around the concept of soft tone of face to symbolic work often helps parents slow down enough to become curious about the more vulnerable feelings that may be projected as anger. Even when a child has been physically safe for a period of time, they may have a hard time experiencing felt safety. Clinicians may be working on two fronts at the same time: (1) helping parents become more aware of their own facial expressions and learn how to soften them and (2) equipping the hurt children in their care to ask for reassurance when they need it. Many of the adoptive parents I work with, as well as the parents of anxious biological children, have the experience of being lost in thought while driving a child home from school. Once the child learns that it is acceptable to ask for reassurance, he may say, "Mommy, you look mad. Are you mad?" Sometimes he will even risk asking, "Are you mad at me?" We train parents to respond with something like this: "Oh, buddy, thanks for letting me know that my expression was confusing to you. I'm not mad at all right now. I was just deep in thought about a work problem I'm trying to solve." Clinicians talk so much with parents about serve-and-return exchanges of communication in building healthy brains. However, parents and clinicians alike tend to focus these exchanges on verbal communication. When a baby smiles and we smile back, this is a serve-and-return communication. The mirror neurons in our brains are meant to engender shared experiences during interpersonal interactions. So, when a parent smiles and a baby smiles in response, the baby is not simply reflexively lifting the corners of his mouth—literally tightening the correct muscles to make a smile—but is most likely experiencing a surge of dopamine and oxytocin that mirrors the neurochemical experience of the parent. The parent and infant are sharing an experience of delight. If neurobiological responses can truly be shared this way, then the implications for soft tone of face become even more important in our exchanges with escalated children. It is likely that our mirror neurons will respond to their upset expressions and internal state with an innate attempt to match them.

I am reminded of a moment in the waiting room of Nurture House some years ago. An 8-year-old child adopted from Ethiopia had, according to Mom, "thrown a fit" on the way to our appointment. The little girl was curled up in a ball, with her face pressed into the fabric of the bench. I approached her from the side and used a soft tone of voice to say hello and then, "Your body is letting me know that you are having a hard time right now. Mom, can you help me understand what has happened?" Mom was exasperated and sitting stiffly with a clenched jaw. I listened and by degrees helped Mom come to the understanding that her daughter had been anticipating getting to jump in a rented bounce house as part of a special celebration in her afterschool program and had not remembered this appointment until she was about to be picked up. The child's posture became more relaxed as I narrated her potential disappointment, confusion, and difficulty verbalizing any of this to her mom. I asked the client if she would risk letting me see her face, and she shook her head violently back and forth while her face remained buried in the cushion. Then I said, "My eyes are soft for you." She peeked at me through her fingers as her mom started to cry. During my next session with the parent, Mom talked about how profound that moment had been for her, and how much she had been reflecting on the hardness or softness of her expression as she worked to create felt safety for her daughter.

When parents are healthy, trusting co-parents—when they genuinely like each other and are on the same team—some of the softness of face work can be done together with both. I have had multiple parents tease the other about the unibrow they get when angry. If there is safety in the relationship, co-parents can be accurate and helpful allies in assisting each other soften their tone of face.

Organize

This first "O" in SOOTHE stands for "organize" and refers to both organizing the child's external environment and organizing the child's internal experience. During the intake, we often ask parents to describe the child's morning routine and/or bedtime routine. Every so often, the prompt "Tell me about your bedtime routine" is met with absolute silence, followed by "You know, we try to get the kids to bed around 9." This serves as a red flag to us that this family will need more help in creating routines and enforcing a schedule than other families might. Sometimes the lack of goodness of fit between a parent and child involves an anxious child and a parent who flies by the seat of his pants. Parents can be supported in providing more structure for the child who needs it, and the more fun we can make it, the easier it will be for both. Sometimes parents need support to reflect on and then tweak the current morning and evening routines. When parents tell us, during the intake, that the mornings are an absolute mess, we begin helping them work through the current morning routine.

A parent may explain that her child gets up at 7 and watches TV while eating breakfast, but then when it is time for him to put on his clothes and shoes, he ignores the parent or ends up in a complete meltdown. In this case, all that may be needed is some rearranging of the schedule: Clothes go on first, as do shoes; then breakfast can be eaten while watching TV. In some families, screens may need to be removed entirely from the morning routine. In other families, screen time may begin once the child is in the car with his backpack and may consist of two funny and short YouTube clips on the way to school. One playful way to help parents—or parents and children together—concretize the schedule is to create a personalized board game for the family. This can be done in session with the clinician's support. Some families will benefit from the support of a blank paper template for a board game, and we have created one (see Figure 5.2) that begins with waking up and ends with going to sleep. This handout can be copied as many times as needed, and children may request their own copies as the schedule is being designed. The goal, however, is toward a personalized schedule for the child that the whole family (including the child) can embrace. Other families will want to create their own winding path of spaces together. Some families enjoy choosing an old board game from home, like Chutes and Ladders or Sorry, and repurposing it. Some families will want to outline the schedule for their whole day within the spaces, and others will focus on just the most problematic part of the day. Figure 5.3 is a board game that was created to help a child get through the morning routine.

Another fun part of the process can involve each family member creating their own game piece. For anyone who has ever played Monopoly, certain game pieces are preferred (my favorite is the top hat) and can engender competition over who will get the most coveted pieces. At Nurture House, we bring the family into the art room, where many materials are displayed in jars at eye level for children and many others are easily accessible in the cabinets with the parent's help. Here, we let the family use any of the materials available to create their own game piece. Organized chaos normally ensues, and the whole exercise can function as a projective activity. Negotiating which family member designs which kind of game piece can be very instructive, both around how the family members cooperate, make decisions, or share resources, and also in how each member wants to be seen or represented in game piece form (see Figure 5.4).

Building Board Games Together

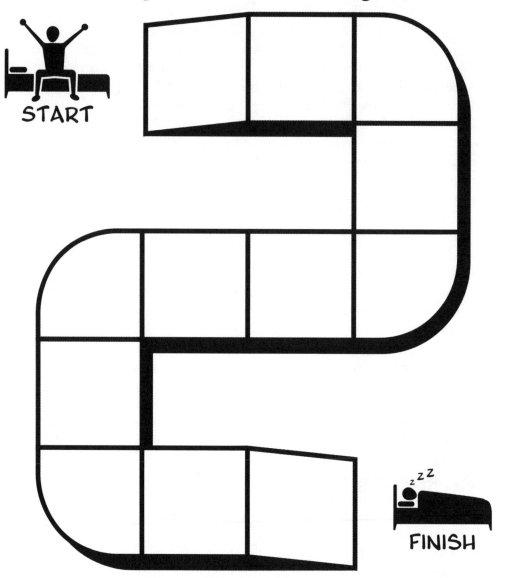

Create a schedule with the board game template above. Work through your child's day, space by space, from wake-up to bedtime, writing in words or drawing pictures to represent breakfast, teeth brushing, reading, screen time, etc. When possible, invite your child to help create it. Have fun coloring it in together.

FIGURE 5.2. Board Game Template for the Schedule.

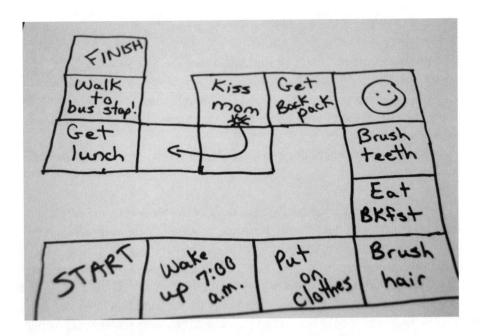

FIGURE 5.3. Example of Child's Morning Schedule.

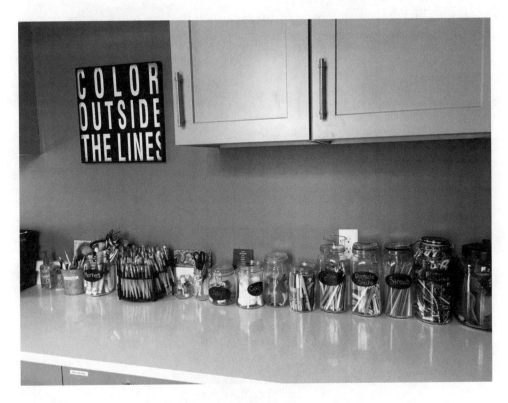

FIGURE 5.4. Creative Space for Families.

Prompts for game piece description could include:

1. Family members design themselves as superheroes.
2. Family members choose an animal to represent themselves and create that symbol.
3. Each family member designs a kind of hat to be their game piece and creates that symbol.

The game board intervention explored above can provide a fun way to encode the various pieces of a busy family schedule or a child's full-day schedule for the family to support, but many times individual children, especially those who struggle with anxiety, can benefit from a reminder schedule that stays with them throughout the day. Some children benefit from personalized schedules. These can be created in a variety of ways, and many basic templates for creating schedules are available online. We keep sets of colorful cut-out people and binder rings on hand. Whenever a child seems to be really struggling with her daily routines, we help her design a pictorial schedule that can be hooked onto her backpack at school, or even onto her belt loop if necessary (see Figure 5.5).

If the child deals with separation anxiety, then the concrete schedule can give the child a transitional object that continues to link her with the parent even when

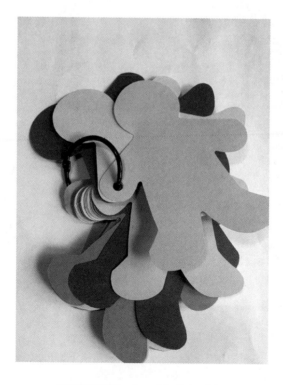

FIGURE 5.5. Portable Schedule.

the child is at school and the parent is at home. The session during which we create the rotating card set includes both parent and child. At the end of the session, the parent is given some extra cut-out people cards to personalize and intersperse among the schedule cards—with notes like "You are half-way through your school day. Good job sticking with it!" or "You have one more hour of school, then I will pick you up and we'll snuggle!" or "Can't wait to see you!" These personalized cards can be traded to provide novelty for the child and to help maintain interest in this personalized pictorial schedule.

New Experiences (the Ultimate Transitions)

Another issue that often comes up, especially with adoptive parents, has to do with how to introduce children to new experiences. Many of the families we work with at Nurture House have adopted a child internationally. These children may come into the home from a hard place, in which they had very few resources, to a luxurious bedroom and possibly even a fully equipped playroom or bonus room. These children are often also signed up for a soccer team or another organized sports team in order to "give them new experiences." The thing is, it requires several honed skills sets for a child to be successful in a team environment. I am thinking of a 7-year-old boy who was adopted internationally at age 3. He had sensory processing issues and delays in his physical, cognitive, emotional, and social development, and he is still playing catch-up at age 7. He responded to his first soccer practice with a flight response, running back to the car. He responded to his first soccer game with a death-feigning response, in which he curled up in the fetal position under the team bench and remained immovable for a period of time. So, what might be needed to help a child who has sensitive neurophysiology for any reason (early neglect or maltreatment, *in utero* exposure to toxins, neurodevelopmental disorders) prepare for a soccer team? The child in question might need to watch some soccer games on TV. The child in question might need to put on his shin guards and wear them around the house to get used to the discomfort brought on by this uncomfortable new sensation. The child might need to put on the cleats and walk around in them in the front yard, experiencing the way in which they sink into the grass. The child might need to learn the rules of the game, meet the coach, meet some of his teammates, or kick the ball around in the front yard with a parent before experiencing a soccer practice—in which the weather, the coach, the teammates, the ball, the rules, and the equipment all have to be navigated. Many parents would perceive this as overkill and think that we may be advocating "babying" behavior. Our "pull yourself up by your bootstraps culture" may be even more toxic for this child, but on some level, yes, I am promoting "babying" behavior—if by this one means returning to early developmental stages and giving a child experiences that were missed in order to provide the scaffolding of neural wiring needed to be ready to expand his microcosm to include team sports.

Another example of the organize strategy is often assessed during the Nurture House Dyadic Assessment (NHDA). There is a task, almost a crescendo of the assessment, that says, "Adult leaves the room for 1 minute without the child." This task was adopted from the Marschak Interaction Method (MIM), the Theraplay assessment tool (Booth & Jernberg, 2010), but hails ultimately from the Strange Situation experiments first completed by Mary Main (Ainsworth & Bell, 1970). We have observed thousands of parents completing this task, and their ways of approaching it vary tremendously. One of my favorite navigations of this task involves a mother first reading the task out loud (which provides a certain degree of structure all by itself) and then, upon seeing her son respond with intense anxiety, saying, "I know . . . you can count to 60 while I'm gone and then I'll come right back in." The child in question clung to Mom's idea and began to count out loud. He regulated himself in this way while his mother listened at the door and returned just as he had counted to 60. This client had experienced a wave of anxiety when faced with being in the playroom without the co-organizing presence of his mother. She correctly interpreted his panic and gave him a developmentally appropriate, rhythmic, structure task (counting out loud) to complete until she returned. This was a fairly sophisticated response to the task. I have had many other parents who read the card somehow feel as if they are not supposed to tell the child what the card says, so they make up a reason to leave, saying they need to use the restroom or check their voicemail. Some dyads find it impossible to navigate the task; the child becomes upset, clinging to the parent, and the parent chooses to stay in the room with the child. With most dyads, the parent is able to successfully exit the room. That's when things get really interesting. The child sometimes handles the parent's absence by sitting quietly in one place, pretending that the therapist is not in the room and awaiting the parent's return. Other children handle the task by immediately jumping up, asking permission to play with certain toys, and engaging with the therapist as another co-regulator while the parent is gone. Still others jump up and occupy themselves with toys but never interact with the therapist in the room.

In live trainings, I often show a video clip of a young man, adopted from Russia at 1 year, who becomes profoundly immobilized when his mother leaves the room. At 7, he sits for a solid minute in a frozen state, barely breathing. When his mother returns, saying in a singsong chipper voice, "OK! I'm back!," we see him collapse in on himself, taking the first deep breath he has since she left the room. The mother continued to use a singsong voice while moving on to the next task, and she had no idea, until we together watched the video, of how powerfully her sudden absence had affected him. He had lost his co-organizer and went into a state of paralyzing fear until she returned. Ironically, the dyad was requesting treatment for how dysregulated this 9-year-old would become. What Mom realized immediately upon watching the video was that her son needed more structure from her, not less. As she strove to be a "nice mom," she was providing him with frequent moments of incongruence.

When we look at Ed Tronick's work, and the Still Face Experiments, we see babies who become completely disorganized when their parent stops providing the organizing presence they desperately need. I find it impossible to watch clips from the Still Face Experiments without smiling, as the mother is first told simply to play with her baby. There is a camera trained on Mom's face and another camera trained on Baby's face—and our view is often presented on a split screen so we can observe both at once. Mom smiles, and Baby smiles back. Baby coos or makes a high-pitched giggle and Mom responds, either matching or unintentionally co-regulating the excitement of playtime with Mom. Then the researcher tells the mom to blunt her affect, to still her face, so that she is sending no signals, positive or negative, to her baby.

What does the baby do when confronted with the sudden absence of the parent's attuned responding? Well, first the baby tries harder. It looks like the baby is saying, "Oh, you're distracted. Let me get back your attention—remind you of how adorable I am, how much fun I am to play with." The baby giggles louder or coos longer and kicks his arms and legs. If Mom still does not respond, the baby begins to decompensate. The baby may begin to drool, will look away from Mom's face, and possibly stare at the wall. Some babies even lose their bowels as a response to the intense dysregulation brought on when Mom is no longer co-organizing their experience. What we have learned is that a vacuum of feedback is terribly frightening to little ones. The Mom described above needed some help learning how incredibly important her moment-to-moment feedback continued to be for her young son. I understand the surprise that Mom experienced when she realized that one of her superpowers was co-organizing her son. This 9-year-old boy had not come home to her from Russia until he was a year old. He had spent all of his *in utero* development under stress. He had spent the first year of his life in a huge hall with 30 other babies. Only his most aggressive attempts at gaining his caregivers' attention would reward him with any level of attunement. At 9, when he is under stress, including the stress of entering a new space without Mom, he needs her co-organizing presence much more than another 9-year-old who received attuned, nurturing care during their first year of life. The really joyful news of neuroplasticity is that, to some extent, as repetitions of earlier missed experiences are given, neural pathways for first being soothed by the other are laid down more deeply, and eventually, these can lead to pathways for self-soothing.

Offer Choices

Offering choices is a fairly standard structure when parents are giving directions. I will talk first about two ways to structure a two-choice procedure, simply because we haven't introduced this concept thoroughly in the book, but will then explore ways that offering the standard two choices may not be effective for children who are dysregulated. Most children who are in their Choosing Mind will respond well to a series of two choices. Children who come from hard beginnings and are still building trust with their caregivers can react positively to a structure in which two choices are offered: the first choice involves having them put on their shoes by themselves, the second with your support in some way. This set of two choices acknowledges that the child from a hard place may need to become more dependent on the parent for a period of time, and offers doing hard things together as a way to fill the child's trust tank. For children with fairly secure attachments, and who will learn from the outcome of their choice regardless, offering the choice to put their shoes on or experience the natural consequence of not doing so is also reasonable. Most likely, each child in our care will need a combination of two choice prompts over time: some in which an instruction may be given that needs some support from the parent to complete and some in which an instruction is given that a child may simply not want to complete at the time. In the first case, we instruct parents to lift their hand with two fingers raised (as a visual prompt) and say, "You have two choices. You can strap yourself into your car seat, or I can help you to do it." Some children, particularly preschoolers, will sometimes choose immediately to do it on their own, as they are compelled to "do things my own self." In the second case, we still instruct parents to again lift two fingers but this time say, "You have two choices. You can choose to leave your jacket in the car or you can choose to wear it but carry it yourself if you get hot while we are looking at the animals. We will sit with parents in session and troubleshoot some of the child's big behaviors. We help parents work through the decision-making tree around whether or not the child is in his Choosing Mind. And if so, does the child need to be offered a second choice that provides support or offers a natural or logical consequence? The parent writes down potential scenarios on the "Two Choices Handout" (see Figure 5.6). We also send home a printout of multiple two-choice prompts, asking the parents to cut them up and use the prompts throughout the week as hard parenting moments arise (see Figure 5.7).

Parents who have been in the habit of giving a direction, waiting only a second or two before recognizing that the child is not yet starting to obey, and quickly repeating the command may find themselves repeating the same things constantly. They may give a direction four or five times, becoming increasingly frustrated each time they do so, and then erupt in anger and mete out disproportionate consequences. So, the other instruction we give to parents involves offering the two choices with words and gestures and then waiting in a curious posture for a count of 5 in their head (also recommended in PCIT) before doing anything further. Some children just need a few seconds to begin to comply, and once a child has begun to comply, thanking her for choosing the way that she did can help everyone feel appreciated.

PCIT, a dyadic treatment that trains parents in giving good commands and unpacks a two-choice discipline procedure (Hembree-Kigin & McNeil, 2013), endorses the use of gestural cues in offering choices. Mehrabian looked at two separate studies on communication and came up with some startling statistics. Only

TWO CHOICES:
WHEN FOCUS IS ENHANCING ATTACHMENT AND BUILDING TRUST.

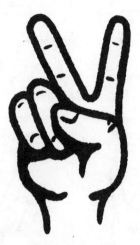

YOU CAN CHOOSE TO _____, OR I CAN HELP YOU TO DO IT.

THE FIRST CHOICE IS DOING THE THING YOU ASKED,
THE OTHER CHOICE IS DOING IT WITH YOUR SUPPORT IN SOME WAY.

TWO CHOICES:
WHEN FOCUS IS LEARNING TO CHOOSE GOOD OUTCOMES.

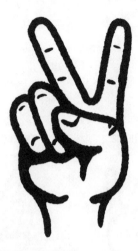

YOU CAN CHOOSE TO _____, OR _____.

THE FIRST CHOICE IS DOING THE THING YOU ASKED,
THE OTHER CHOICE IS A NATURAL CONSEQUENCE OF NOT DOING IT.

FIGURE 5.6. Two Choices Handout.

7% of our communication is made up of the verbal content. Seven percent, wow. PCIT offers a worksheet for parents called "Giving Good Commands." It breaks down about 11 steps to communicating an instruction to a child. These dimensions include things like giving one instruction at a time, making it specific, stating it positively, and remaining polite. The other 93% of communication is broken down into body language (55%) and tone of voice (38%). Now we know that what you say is not nearly as important as how you say it. This is why instructions need to be delivered in a neutral tone of voice. From a trauma-informed lens, even a benign instruction delivered in a harsh tone can arm the fear-based brain of an easily dysregulated child and negatively influence compliance. It can even result in a parasympathetic collapse response or a sympathetic uptick in heart rate, blood pressure, or cortisol release in the traumatized child's physiology.

When I was training a staff of 20 volunteers to become co-regulators for the children at Camp Nurture, I taught them all to lift two fingers when saying, "You

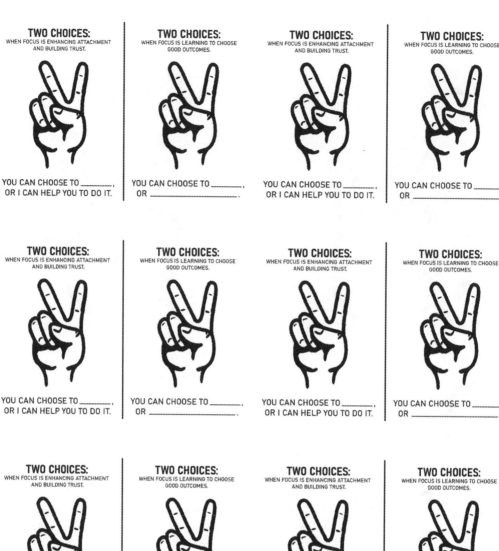

FIGURE 5.7. Two Choices Homework Handout.

have two choices" Since 55% of our communication is nonverbal, the use of a gestural cue can dramatically enhance the power of what you are saying, while also giving the child a focal point for visual attention. Moreover, it helps to structure the parent or clinician who is offering the choices, and (between you and me) gives the grown-up a moment's breathing room to decide what the two choices should be! One of our senior staff, a seasoned counselor in her own right, admitted that using the two-choice procedure was challenging for her. She reported that, as she would lift her fingers in a semicircle and say the words, "You have two choices," her brain would be screaming, "What the heck are they?" This feeling resonated so deeply with the staff that we had T-shirts made: On the front is the prompt "You have two choices," and on the back "What the heck are they?" It is important to remember that parents are learning a new way to communicate, in the middle of sometimes stressful situations with children who are not following directions. The cartoon in Figure 5.8 can be shared with parents as a humorous way of acknowledging that we are often figuring out the two choices as we go.

Sometimes, however, even two choices is one too many. I will tell on myself here. When my oldest son was 7, I homeschooled him 3 days a week, and he was in a homeschool co-op for the 2 days I saw clients. He was a fairly anxious child (in fact, I wrote the Worry Wars curriculum with him in mind), and one day my sessions ended early and I thought it would be tons of fun to surprise him at school, have him dismissed early, and take him out on a special Mommy–Son date. I showed up at school a half-hour before the day was over, which flustered him somewhat as he didn't have time to pack up his backpack according to the classroom routines. However, he rallied, and when we got out to the car and he was strapped in, I turned to him with excitement in my eyes and said, "Guess what? You and I get to have a superspecial date today. We can go see the new *Tooth Fairy* movie or we can go bowling. Which would you rather do? It was like watching the unwieldy weight and shape of planet earth descend on his little shoulders. For 45 minutes, he wrestled in this way with the two choices: "Well, if we go to see the movie and it's not very good, we will have missed out on our chance to go bowling. But if we go bowling, and I'm not very good at it, we will have missed out on the movie." I had set him up for actually experiencing more pressure from the two choices offered than he would have experienced if I had just showed up and told him the plan. In fairness to us both, we still would have weathered an adjustment period of probably 15 minutes or so, in which he would have been coming to terms with the change from his normal schedule, because even if the change was due to something new or exciting, it would still be change. The upshot of this story is that sometimes the most soothing strategy is to offer only one choice and allow it time to sink in.

There is another scenario that is equally dysregulating for some children, especially those who have significant amounts of early adverse childhood experiences. Remember that early trauma impacts the functioning of our reptilian brain stem, our diencephalon, and our limbic brain, and potentially compromises the integrity of lower brain region scaffolding as it is meant to support executive functioning

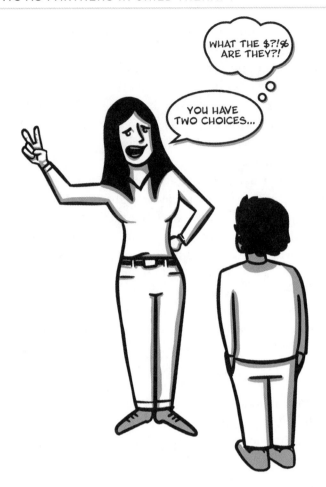

FIGURE 5.8. Two Choices: What the Heck Are They?

skills, such as decision making. When children without enough neuro-scaffolding are asked to make a choice between an overwhelming number of options, their arousal systems may kick them into "fight, flight, and freeze" or collapse. This was the case for Danny. Danny had endured sexual abuse, physical abuse, and intense neglect for the first 4 years of his life. He was removed from his biological home and placed with an adoptive parent who worked fiercely on his behalf to provide experiences of health for him. Together, Danny and his adoptive mother had made great strides in creating safety and trust in their relationship, and Danny's worst behaviors had subsided significantly. Mom reported that he was having "full-blown meltdowns" only once or twice a month. I asked if she could gather some baseline data about when and where these were happening, and when she returned, she was smiling in a slightly self-deprecating way as she said, "I think I figured it out. The meltdowns happen mainly when we go to the Super Walmart to do our weekly grocery shopping trip." Mom explained that she had been implementing all the strategies we had practiced together. She was keeping him close, giving him clearly defined jobs, delighting in his help as he returned with the box of cereal or the can of soup. At the end of the very successful, hour-long shopping trip, Mom would say, "Since you did such a great job helping me, let's go to the candy aisle." They would move to the candy aisle, and she would invite him to pick a candy from the multitude of choices. Just for fun one day, I counted the number of candy choices on that aisle of the Super Walmart and I counted at least 50. What Mom had not realized was that he had used up all of his executive functioning abilities during the hour that he was navigating the bright lights, the loud noise, the overstimulation of the environment . . . and that asking him to make what felt like a monumental choice to him without narrowing the field of choices was outside of his Window of Tolerance for stress. On one occasion, the decision was so overwhelming, he curled up in the fetal position on the shelf lowest to the ground, and it took about 15 minutes to get him out again.

Once we realized what the problem was for Danny, we simply tweaked the pattern of executive function use. Mom would talk with her son on the way to the store, offering him a choice between a couple of his favorite candies. He would make the cognitive choice before they even entered the store, and once they walked in, he was free to go ahead and put the Hershey bar or the bag of Reese's Pieces in his pocket. He could anchor himself to the choice by touching the candy in his pocket at any point in the shopping trip, and as soon as they were in the check-out line, he could begin eating it and they would scan the wrapper for payment. Too many choices or too few? The clinician serves as a co-investigator of the needs of the child who is coming for treatment and designs healthy parameters for the child to continue growing their Window of Tolerance for stress without kicking the child into a state of hyper- or hypoarousal.

Offer a Way Out

The other meaning of "offer," as it is encoded in the SOOTHE strategies, has to do with how we offer a way out for children who are stuck in a fight, flight, or freeze response. There is another video that I show frequently when illustrating this concept. Another task from the MIM reads like this, "Adult and child put lotion on each other." A whole host of reasons explain why a child might not actually want to have lotion applied by a parent, including sensory sensitivities, intimacy issues, feeling like the task is for younger children. However, watching how the parent and child navigate this discomfort together is where the real meat of the learning, at least for the clinician who is hoping to intervene in the system, takes place. I shared a vignette earlier in which a mother of a highly anxious child organized his experience in the playroom when she needed to leave by having him count out loud until she returned. This same client was also loathe to have any lotion applied. What follows is a transcript of his interaction with his mom around this task:

MOM: Where do you want your lotion?

PAUL (*with a scowl on his face and a challenge in his voice*): Hair!

MOM: (*laughing*) No . . . (*while rubbing the lotion between her hands to warm it*) can I put some on your skin?

PAUL: (*in a shrill, whiny voice*) Noooo.

MOM: You don't like that?

PAUL: (*Shakes his head vigorously "no."*)

MOM: Would you like it anywhere on your sk . . . on your body?

PAUL: No! Just my hair.

MOM: (*rubbing the lotion into her own skin*) Well, I can't really put lotion in your hair, and you know what, I'm remembering about you that you don't like lotion. Can I just rub this stuff in real quick (*rubbing the lotion completely into her own arms*)? OK? And I don't have any more lotion on my hands. So, would you like me to just rub your back?

PAUL: (*Looks suspiciously and shakes his head slightly "no."*)

MOM: I can just rub your back, and we can pretend there is lotion. Would you like that?

[Paul moves toward her, giving her his back, but when she goes to touch him, he says "no!" in a panicky tone. Mom reassures him, saying, "There is nothing on my hand. Totally nongreasy—so I can just rub your back." Paul allows her to rub his back, although his face remains tense.]

MOM: Rub your back . . . and then maybe after I've rubbed your back for a minute, you can put some lotion on me. Does that feel good (*her voice infused with nurture*)? Is there any other place you'd like to be rubbed?

PAUL: (*whispering*) Just my back.

MOM: (*whispering in response*) Just your back? (*still whispering*) Do you want to lie down so you're comfortable?

PAUL: (*after lying on her lap for a few seconds*) Now I'll put some on you.

Showing this clip in live trainings has sometimes been a mixed bag. Behaviorally oriented clinicians will often say, "Well, she didn't make him do the task at all. She let him walk all over her." I always find this response bewildering, because the whole interaction feels like a moment of really attuned co-regulation by a Safe Boss parent of her highly anxious and dysregulated child. If she had insisted that he allow his arm or hand to be lotioned, he would have tipped over the edge into a full-blown meltdown. She felt how very close to the edge he was and said, "I'm remembering about you that you don't like lotion." "I'm remembering about you" is a power-ful turn of phrase. She is communicating to him that she is his Storykeeper—she knows him better than anyone else. She knows what he likes and what he doesn't like. She can see past the dug-in "no!" to a solution to the problem; she offers him a way out. I find this a beautiful example of Mom's ability to co-regulate her son.

If, when the child in our care crosses his arms in front of his chest and says, "No, I won't!!" we can put on our SuperParent goggles and see, at this moment of rebellion, that the child is 6 feet deep in a clay-packed hole (see Figure 5.9.), then we can see that he has no way out, without the grown-up involved.

One child, while reflecting on his dug-in behavior from the week before, took this small digging man and trapped him within four walls that were as tall as he was (see Figure 5.10). This child went on to talk about feeling like he just kept making the hole deeper.

In these hard moments, it is up to the grown-up to throw in a ladder or build a staircase. The child or teen is not able to pull herself out of the hole; she needs her Safe Boss to help. Do you remember any time in your own childhood when you became so entrenched in a decision that you couldn't get yourself out of it? I remember vividly more than one occasion, as a teenager, when I had behaved in a snarky way with my mom. I remember her saying, "Why can't you just apologize?," but I was so dug in to my own "NO" that I couldn't see a way out of it. I didn't know why I couldn't apologize, I just couldn't. When Paul got completely dug in to his "NO" regarding lotion, this mother found a work-around. She first set herself up as his Storykeeper and then offered, from that role, another path to accomplishing the same end. How do we offer the dug-in child a way out? A Safe Boss throws in a ladder. The dug-in child cannot get himself out, but needs his Safe Boss to make a way (see Figure 5.11). We work with parents to determine what alternative ways out there might be for the child.

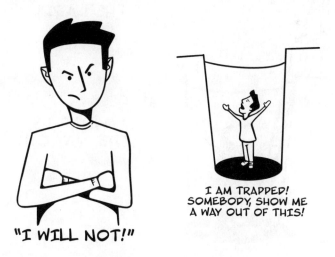

"I WILL NOT!"

I AM TRAPPED!
SOMEBODY, SHOW ME
A WAY OUT OF THIS!

FIGURE 5.9. Six-Feet Deep.

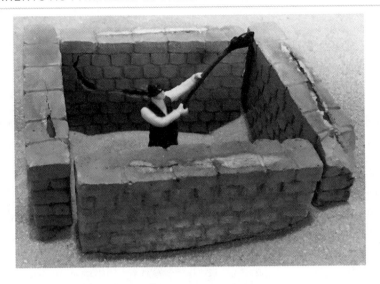

FIGURE 5.10. In a Hole.

Touch and Physical Proximity

Many of you have seen the iconic picture of the two twin preemies, sisters who became the guinea pigs for changing the way that neonatal nursing works. In the 1970s, twin girls were born 12 weeks premature at the Medical Center of Central Massachusetts. At that time, there was no protocol for putting babies together in incubators, so each baby was being taken care of separately. One baby was doing well, but the other was having trouble regulating. Her heart rate and body temperature

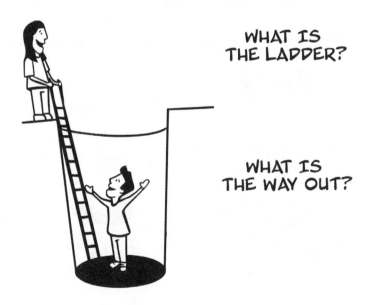

FIGURE 5.11. What Is the Way Out?

were erratic, and her vitals were tanking. The pioneering nurse in charge of the Neonatal Intensive Care Unit at that time broke protocol and, purely on instinct, placed the stronger of the two sisters in the same incubator as her sibling. Almost immediately, the sister threw her arm over her sibling, and within minutes the other sibling's vitals began to regulate. Touch. Connection. Primal needs that precede experience, education, or even consciousness.

Touch can be an extremely regulating tool, especially when a child is sensory seeking and benefits from more sensory input. While we can provide children with therapeutic experiences that involve touch, facilitating the therapeutic use of healthy touch between parents and children enhances these most important attachment relationships, while mitigating clinician's concerns that touching children may open them up to malpractice risks. I often speak at maltreatment conferences that are attended by law enforcement, Department of Child Services workers, forensic interviewers, judges, and therapists for children who have experienced sexual abuse, physical abuse, or extreme neglect. When I began speaking at these conferences, there would always be one person in the audience who would raise her hand and then begin to ask about the risks of retraumatizing a child who has been sexually abused by touching him in any way. I welcomed the question, as it gave me an opportunity to begin shifting the paradigm for our helping community. The short answer is this: I don't know anyone who needs good, safe, nurturing touch more than a child who has been sexually abused. If sexualized touch is the only kind of touch that a child has received, as is often the case with children who have been sexually abused and otherwise neglected, then this child is unlikely to have developed a capacity to discern the difference between good, safe, nurturing touch and inappropriate touch. We talk about this discernment as the "warning bell in your head" or the "uh-oh button in your stomach" (Goodyear-Brown, 2013). Children who have received lots of good, safe, nurturing touch have an uh-oh button and recognize a feeling of discomfort when a touching boundary has been violated.

When I first encountered this phenomenon, the pigeon-holing of touch as a dangerous practice in working with traumatized children, I went in search of a metaphor to help shift professional paradigms. I have an FBI agent to thank for introducing me to the one I now use. At a multidisciplinary conference, I was seated next to him; he had completed several undercover sting operations with regard to human trafficking. We talked at length about that and then I ask about counterfeit money, a topic that has always fascinated me. I said, "So, how do all the FBI agents stay up to speed on the new forms of counterfeit money? Do you have seminars on each new kind? Does someone send an email to all the agents with pictures of counterfeits as they are discovered?" He laughed at me a little and said, "No. Actually, we don't spend any time with counterfeit money. In our trainings, we spend all of our time with real dollar bills. We hold them up to the light, we feel the weight of them in our hands, we even taste them. We get to know them so well that when we come across a phony, we just know it." Do you hear the parallel between this training to identify counterfeit money and the training of children to identify counterfeit touch? When children have lots and lots of experiences of healthy touch, they just know a phony touch when they feel it.

The benefits of healthy touch in the healthy development of children are well documented (Courtney, 2014; Dunbar, 2010; Field, Diego, & Hernandez-Reif, 2007; Field et al., 1986, 2019), yet many clinicians are hesitant to use touch in therapy (McKinney & Kempson, 2012). Touch is important in facilitating attachments (Bowlby, 1969, 1988); in moving from co-regulation to self-regulation (Feldman & Eidelman, 2007); in developing boundaries; and in learning where your body ends and another's begins. I realize that the following description may be overly simplistic, but it is a good starting place for most of the parents and teachers that we train. We show the image of a child in full-blown tantrum mode and say, "This is cortisol." We go on to explain that when children are in significant distress, cortisol, the stress hormone, is released in massive quantities into their little bodies. Next, we show a picture of two chimpanzees snuggling together and say, "If that was cortisol, then this is oxytocin." We go on to explain that oxytocin is the bonding chemical. It is released in the brains of both mother and infant when they are nursing. It is also released through other forms of nurturing touch, through humor, and through play. If cortisol, released in massive amounts, is toxic to the developing systems of a child, then oxytocin is the antidote . . . or at least part of it (Thompson, Callaghan, Hunt, Cornish, & McGregor, 2007; Uvnäs-Moberg & Francis, 2003). I talk about this often in relation to the playroom, labeling the fully equipped playroom and an attuned play therapist as a neurochemical boxing ring. When working with parents, we want them to understand the superpowers they possess as caregivers, so they can use the yummy neurochemical cocktail that their nurturing touch provides to help with regulation and connection.

Touch can also provide an important anchor for a child who needs to focus their cognitive energies. I have written previously about Camp Nurture, the intensive day camp that our team offered for highly dysregulated adopted children and their parents. Buddies and back-up buddies were trained to attune to the needs of the child in their care. The internal disorganization of these children and their resulting big behaviors required us to narrow the focus of work for the week to enhancing regulation and connection. I did not expect prolonged focused attention, as we were working to lay down new and deeper neural pathways in the reptilian brain stem and the limbic brain. We were not focused on the thinking brain or on executive function. I did not even attempt to read a book to the group on the first 2 days of camp, but decided to begin the book *How Are You Peeling?* on Day 3. I was fully prepared to be interrupted by dysregulated behavior within the first few pages and was prepared to say, "Your bodies are letting me know that you need to get your bodies moving!" I read the first three pages to the group and kept on reading. I ended up finishing the book and was a little dumbfounded as to how this had happened—until I saw a photo taken of the reading session. Look at Figure 5.12 and see if you can figure out what all three children pictured have in common. What do you see?

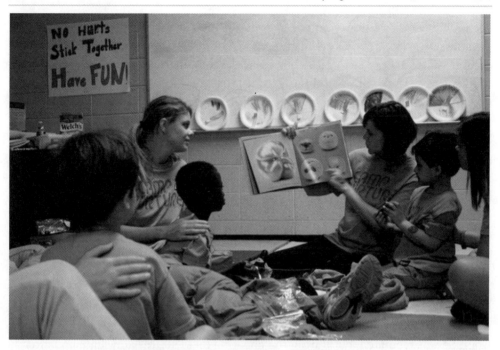

FIGURE 5.12. Anchoring Children through Supportive Touch.

Each of the buddies has her hand on the back of her assigned child. I had engaged in many hours of training with our buddies, but at no time had I said, "Be sure to put your hand on your child's back during storytime." I wouldn't have thought to encourage this. I simply taught them how to attune to the needs of the child in their care. It seems that these three children needed the anchor of touch to free up their cognitive capacities to focus on the story.

The addition of physical proximity as an alternative to physical touch reflects that while many children are anchored or regulated by touch, a subset of children are triggered or escalated by touch, especially if they are already feeling armed or under threat. It is important that our clinical assessments reflect the nuance of when touch is a help and when it is a hindrance. When I worked in the inner-city schools of Nashville, I completed multiple Functional Behavior Assessments (FBAs) for children with behavioral spikes in an effort to develop individualized Positive Behavior Support Plans (PBSPs). In many cases, these children had experienced or were still experiencing physical abuse, corporal discipline, or domestic violence in their homes. I developed one such FBA for Derrick, a 7-year-old second grader with a very short fuse, who was constantly getting into trouble in his classroom. As you read this series of events, you will begin to see that the teacher continually made choices to further escalate the situation. One morning, Derrick was taking a spelling test with the rest of his classmates. His teacher, we'll call her Miss Ross, was sitting at her desk at the front of the room when she noticed Derrick cheating. She called him out in front of the class, saying sharply, "Derrick, I see you cheating. Please go throw your paper away." What's she doing? She's escalating the situation. Who holds the keys to the gradebook? She does. She could have simply chosen not to record his grade, but instead she embarrassed him in front of his classmates. Derrick got up and sauntered across the room slowly and then dangled the paper over the trash can, giving his teacher a look like "You gonna make me?" Miss Ross got up and walked to him across the room. What's she doing? She's escalating the situation. She says with a tight smile on her face, "I said to please put the paper in the trash." He stood looking at her for another few seconds. Later she reported that she "gently placed" her hand on his back to "help him" throw away the paper. He whirled around with his fist raised. He did not hit her, which I considered to show remarkable restraint for my client, and she took him down into a full-body restraint. He was suspended for 10 days, and during the official suspension hearing, the school was seriously entertaining the possibility of expelling him and having him repeat second grade next year. However, when we looked together at the FBA, a clear recommendation had been written into it: This student was *not* to be touched during moments of discipline. To be clear, it was not prohibited—it was even encouraged—for Derrick to receive high fives, fist bumps, and hello hugs when he was regulated, but during the cheating incident, his amygdala had already been armed. It was a ramp-up. In this case, the "gentle touch" on his back triggered escalation.

When physical touch is known to be a trigger, attachment figures can still stay close, maintaining physical proximity as a way to bring regulation and focus when needed. For example, in a classroom two students are whispering to each other while the teacher is giving a social studies lesson. The teacher can choose to interrupt her teaching to say, "Hey, you guys, eyes on me. Pay attention, please." She might have to do this multiple times, interrupting her own focus and that of the other students. If instead she slowly moves closer, walking as she speaks, until her physical body is much closer to the desks of the two boys misbehaving, her physical proximity is likely to interrupt and refocus the boys without her ever looking at them.

Hear the Underlying Anxiety

The "H" in the SOOTHE acronym is for "hear the underlying anxiety." When children's anxiety is spiked, they often dig in for control. Certainly, many of the children who are seen in therapy enter therapy with a control foundation. When asked to do something that makes them anxious, they may respond with "NO!," which ostensibly sounds like defiance. However, there is often a river of anxiety running underneath it. The parent who is bigger, stronger, wiser, and kind is always working to discern when a child is saying "no" from a will-based posture and when a child is saying "no" as a way to cope with underlying anxiety. This is no easy task. Let's say you are taking care of two children. They have taken off their shoes to run around the bonus room together. When it is time to go, you say, "Hey, it's time to put your shoes on." They both say "no." One of the children may be saying "no" because she simply doesn't want to stop playing. The other child may be really saying, "I don't really know how to tie my shoes yet and it makes me feel incompetent to try." If you are able to hear the underlying anxiety, you can use the moment to actually enhance your position as Safe Boss and Storykeeper for the child by saying, "I'm remembering about you that you are learning to tie your shoes. Please put your shoes on your feet and I will help you to tie them."

Parents have often been taught that if they give a direction or a command, they have to stick to it no matter what. This is not the case. For years, I have been trying to come up with a metaphor to help parents shift their paradigm in this way. I believe that it just makes us good assessors of the environment—in other words, it makes us good leaders—to be able to recognize when a command we have given is just too much or too hard for right now. Recently, however, I have been introduced to the Waze app. It's awesome and has gained popularity so quickly because it monitors traffic patterns moment to moment. As a driver, I have a destination and a series of directions on how to get there. I am eating up the roadway as I speed down 65 North when all of a sudden Waze tells me that there is a wreck up ahead. The crash has just occurred, but already traffic is backed up for a mile, and Waze is giving me an alternative route. In a traffic app, we consider this the height of sophistication, but we are likely to perceive similarly flexible changes in directions given by parents as inconsistent. Parents may need lots of permission, reassurance, and practice to take in the lay of the land and begin offering alternative routes, compromises, and revised directions when following the direction as stated may just be too difficult for the child. Figure 5.13 is a handout meant to help parents make this shift. Once we have given the parent this handout, we ask that he spend the week looking for a parenting situation in which he can reroute his direction for a better outcome. We ask that he bring in this example for our next parent coaching session. With multiple practical applications and the support of the therapist, parents can shift their paradigms to seeing rerouting as a strength instead of a weakness.

End and Let Go

The "E" in the SOOTHE acronym stands for "end and let go." Ending an escalation with a child can be hard in the best of circumstances. When I worked in the therapeutic preschool in our local community mental health center, the children would escalate often to the point of having to be physically restrained. Counselors were certified yearly in crisis intervention, verbal de-escalation, and safe physical restraint procedures. We were taught that once the child was physically safe in a restraint, we should repeat the statement "When your body is safe, I will let you go." However, what we found in application was that if the child's body was calm but she was still all riled up on the inside—as evidenced sometimes by her body

AN AERIAL VIEW TO GIVING DIRECTIONS

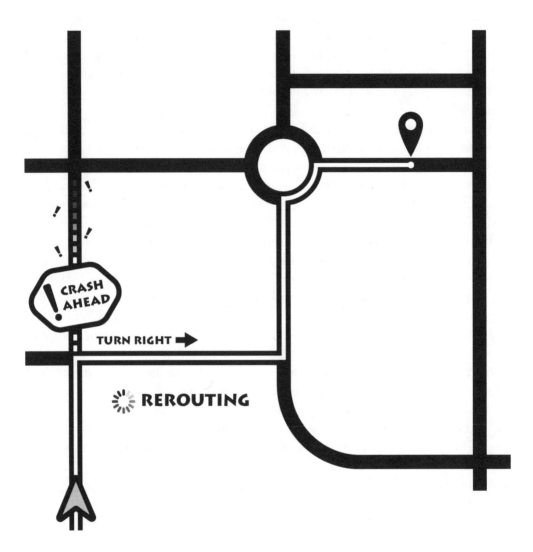

FIGURE 5.13. Finding an Alternate Course Can Be Wise.

being very rigid and her breathing very shallow or quick, or her mumbling obsceni-ties under her breath—once we let go of the child, she would ramp back up within the hour, become aggressive to the point where she needed to be restrained again, and the vicious cycle would continue. We also found that if we gave it more time, and continued to regulate and connect with the child, eventually moving from a hold to a hug or another nurturing interaction, she would de-escalate fully and we wouldn't see the big behaviors again for the rest of the day. I have often wondered if those tiny humans, who had already experienced so much aggression from others and spent so much of their time afraid and armed for danger, were asking for a con-nection in the only way they knew how. The upshot of the "end" in SOOTHE is to help parents identify when a child is well and truly back to baseline, which may often require the investment of another few minutes of the parent's time beyond putting out the fire of the moment.

The second aspect of the "end and let go" has to do with how a parent moves past a blowup. Some of the children we see have the stress/anxiety/anger/energy (insert whichever word makes sense to the parent) build up, and build up somati-cally, to the point where they almost have to explode. Once they have blown up, they feel better. They may have reestablished equilibrium. However, all that upset energy is now in the air. The images shown here, drawn by an adolescent client many years ago, illustrate this point dramatically. In the first picture, he experiences the mounting pressure inside of him as a tornado in his stomach (see Figure 5.14). The second picture depicts how much happier he feels after he has blown up, but the discharged energy is now in the environment (see Figure 5.15).

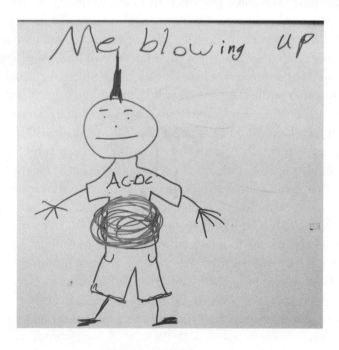

FIGURE 5.14. Mad Inside.

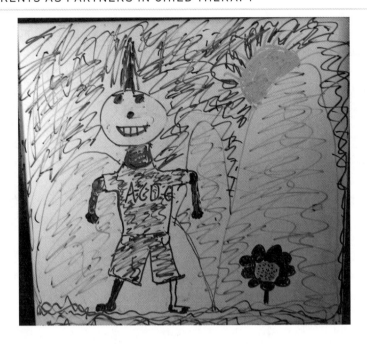

FIGURE 5.15. Mad Released.

When a child has destroyed property, kicked, screamed, scratched, or otherwise escalated, the parent who has been dealing with the storm is probably exhausted. However, when a child is de-escalating from an upset is sometimes the moment when they are most vulnerable and open to new learning. The parents, however, may feel like they need a time-out for themselves. For many of our clients, just after an upset is the most important time for staying close, but the parent may ask for space or distance so that each of them can regroup. We have developed a short list of books that we ask parents to keep on hand, so after an escalation, the parent and child can sit together while the parent reads the book out loud. The books include titles such as the following: *This Is the House That Jack Built* by Sims Taback (2009); *Brown Bear, Brown Bear, What Do You See?* by Bill Martin Jr. (1997); *The Napping House* by Audrey Wood (2015); and *There Was an Old Lady Who Swallowed a Fly!* by Lucille Colandro (2014). This list is not exhaustive but is meant to give examples of books that have a comforting cadence and soothe the reptilian brain stem through rhythmic repetition. Have you ever read a picture book out loud to a child while part of your brain is thinking about something else? So have I. This strategy does not require the parent to have returned already to optimal levels of arousal, but can offer a structured path for parent and child maintaining close physical proximity while regulating together. Clinicians will want to encourage parents not to give any consequences or attempt to discipline further until at least one book has been read, so everyone has had time to bring their thinking brains a little bit more online.

The SOOTHE strategies are not rocket science, but they do serve as an easily absorbed rubric for caregiving behaviors that can help to regulate the lower brain regions of our children and teens when they are escalated. Clinicians will need to use their clinical wisdom in matching the pace of psychoeducation with the needs and capacity of the family system. Some parents present with a desire to absorb information, are high achievers in their own right, and will immediately work to implement any new tool that you offer. Other parents may need to be taught just one SOOTHE strategy at a time, followed up with lots of support, including *in vivo* practice and specialized, easily achievable homework assignments. Two handouts are offered here. The first is a shorthand copy of the SOOTHE strategies that can be printed out and given to parents as a reminder of the skills sets they need (Figure 5.16). The homework sheet offered in Figure 5.17 was created to help parents try out and track their caregiving behaviors once they have been introduced to all the SOOTHE strategies.

SOOTHE!

S = soft tone of voice and face

O = organize

O = offer

T = touch and physical proximity

H = hear the underlying anxiety

E = end and let go

FIGURE 5.16. SOOTHE Handout.

S Soft Tone of Voice	**O** Organize	**O** Offer	**T** Touch	**H** Hear	**E** End
Day: _____ Event:	Day: _____ Event:	Day: _____ Event:	Day: _____ Event:	Day: _____ Event:	Day: _____ Event:
How helpful? _____	How helpful? _____	How helpful? _____	How helpful? _____	How helpful? _____	How helpful? _____
Day: _____ Event:	Day: _____ Event:	Day: _____ Event:	Day: _____ Event:	Day: _____ Event:	Day: _____ Event:
How helpful? _____	How helpful? _____	How helpful? _____	How helpful? _____	How helpful? _____	How helpful? _____
Day: _____ Event:	Day: _____ Event:	Day: _____ Event:	Day: _____ Event:	Day: _____ Event:	Day: _____ Event:
How helpful? _____	How helpful? _____	How helpful? _____	How helpful? _____	How helpful? _____	How helpful? _____

**Please record three moments in the course of the week in which you used a SOOTHE strategy to calm your foster child. Write a few words that will help you remember the event and how the child responded to your intervention. Write in a number by "How helpful" according to the following scale: 1 = Not at all helpful, 2 = A little bit helpful, 3 = Somewhat helpful, 4 = Very helpful, 5 = Extremely helpful.

FIGURE 5.17. SOOTHE Parent Homework Sheet.

CHAPTER 6

Helping Parents Be Fun and Fully Present

Really? Is having fun together important? Yes. Is it attainable? Sometimes. This chapter will highlight the role of delighting in our children and enjoying life with them as primary mitigators of dysregulation and trauma responses. In our current culture, this often requires someone in a clinical or coaching role to help parents make room for fun in the daily or weekly schedule—cultivating delight with great intentionality. As a working mother of three, I sometimes interact with my children with only one part of myself: I may be smiling absentmindedly as they talk while only partially listening to what they are saying, or reading to them while thinking through tomorrow's to-do list. Figure 6.1 presents a powerful sand tray

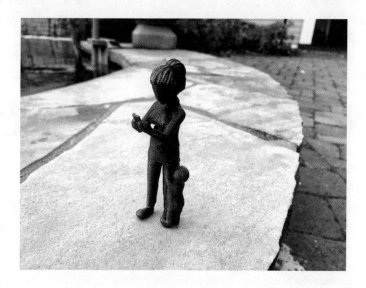

FIGURE 6.1. Distracted Mom.

figure, created on a 3-D printer by Kennedy's Sandplay Mini's. It depicts the modern scenario in which a parent is deeply engaged with their phone while the child is pulling at the parent's leg, begging for attention.

In our current culture, our brains are literally being trained to split attention while moving at breakneck speed throughout our day. Children need time. They need time to sit, without a plan or a diversion, until a creative endeavor emerges. They need empty boxes, masking tape, and leftover oatmeal containers. The most imaginative, creative play often comes after a period of quiet and rest. Part of what we are asking parents to do is to recreate with their children more frequently. *Recreation* is a word that, in modern times, usually refers to entertainment or the passive reception of information-binging Netflix, going to the movies, watching a TED Talk. The root word, *create*, implies action—our active involvement. When we are depleted, we refill ourselves, often in relationship to those closest to us. TraumaPlay therapists begin this process by helping parents and children carve out physical, boundaried space for fun. We call these physical spaces Nurture Nooks. These contained areas for fun and fully present involvement between parent and child help parents focus in on the here and now. I like the mantra, *families that play together stay together* and we know that play can be an important part of helping families heal (Gil, 2014). It is more and more challenging for parents to carve out time for mindful moments with their children or their partners. Play itself, play in relationships, and the neurochemical implications of fun are all mitigators of a family's approach to hard things. Whether the family system is currently experiencing conflict or not, the daily doses of fully present fun in the homemade Nurture Nook protect against harder moments that the family might experience together. Our first Nurture Nook, created in the loft of Nurture House, afforded opportunities for very intimate therapeutic work that would have been difficult to do without the smallness of space (see Figure 6.2). This room has lower ceilings and a small alcove with windows, offering lots of natural light and a view of the trees, while creating clear boundaries as a separate, smaller space in the room.

Clinicians can create Nurture Nooks in their own offices and help parents or teachers design Nurture Nooks that will fit within their unique environments. A Nurture Nook is a space set apart from the rest of a room or building. It should be snug . . . the smallness of the space should communicate the neuroception of safety to a child without making the child or teen feel claustrophobic (Goodyear-Brown, 2019). For many traumatized children, larger spaces encourage hypervigilance, nudging the child on an unconscious level to continue scanning the environment for signs of impending threat. When the environment is made smaller, we communicate to children through their "proprioception" (the way in which their body experiences the world) that they are safe. It is helpful if the Nurture Nook can offer natural light during the day and warm lamp lighting when ambient light is being used to shift the focus of a client's reality to the center of the safe space. At Nurture House, we have a revolving solar-powered crystal that throws magical sparkles across the walls and cushions when a child is in need of a fairytale experience. We

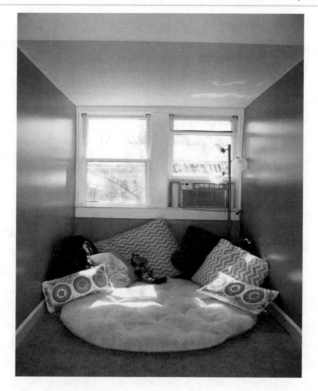

FIGURE 6.2. Nurture House Nook.

recommend having pillows of various kinds of fabric in order to meet a variety of sensory needs and to offer a new sensory experience when a child is needing something novel, but tactile, to remain grounded in the Nurture Nook.

We see many children who spend the majority of their time in a dysregulated state. Asking a parent–child dyad to remain engaged with us in this smaller, intimate space is challenging for some and may require small doses of time spent in the Nurture Nook to help families acclimate. The family's introduction to the Nurture Nook can be titrated, with the first or last few minutes of a session spent here. Once the hypervigilant response has been tempered through the snugness of space, traumatized children can pay attention to more nuanced cues from their partners. Social yet often unconscious exchanges between two people form the building blocks of a relationship. The Nurture Nook is meant to be a place where circles of communication can be opened and closed in rich, satisfying cycles with few distractions. The therapist or the parent becomes the primary toy in the room. It is best for the therapist to provide a lot of structure in the beginning, as a parent and child begin to use the Nurture Nook to enhance their connections to one another, particularly if the child comes from severe trauma or neglect. TraumaPlay therapists talk a great deal about the importance of titration: making sure we provide new experiences for a dyad in doses that are tolerable for both parent and child, allowing them to both experience competence, delight in one another, and enjoy their interactions with the therapist. Play offers a powerful avenue to further connecting humans to one another, based on science, bathed in artistic application, and resulting in almost magical shifts in relationship between parents and children (Kestly, 2015; Porges, 2015; Stewart, Field, & Echterling, 2016; Wheeler & Dillman Taylor, 2016).

I believe that *delight*, as it is fleshed out and communicated concretely to parents and children, is the primary change agent for families to begin healing. By the time most families come to therapy, individual members are often fed up with each other, parents feel exhausted and ineffectual, and children believe that they wield either too much or not enough power or control within the family system. Nurture Nooks are meant to be a facilitated space for a parent and child to enjoy time together, knowing that the safe presence of the therapist will ensure that neither is likely to fail. Sometimes the family system has been so chaotic and children's behaviors have been so out of control that even basic rhythms, like reading books together, have not been established. A child's earliest experiences, those within the first year of life, are, for better or worse, tied to a caregiver and the caregiving patterns experienced in this first year influence development for a lifetime (Sroufe, Coffino, & Carlson, 2010). When children did not get nurturing, attuned care during that first year of life, the Nurture Nook provides a protected space in which children can engage in these kinds of experiences with few distractions and absorb delight, nurture, and care from a Safe Boss. The Nurture Nook is a place that allows parents and children to practice caring for one another, snuggling together, learning together, and communicating safely with each other. We generally encourage families to begin creating their own Nurture Nook—a carved-out space for one-on-one time together—at home only after they have experienced two or three sessions in the therapist's Nurture Nook, guided by the facilitation of the therapist. Taking care of hurts, sharing snacks, reading and snuggling, mirroring games, nurturing dyadic activities, all can happen in the Nurture Nook. Mindfulness work has many beneficial effects for both children and adults (Kabat-Zinn, 2003; Shapiro, Carlson, Astin, & Freedman, 2006; Burke, 2010), and Nurture Nooks invite parents and children to experience mindfulness training together. Not all families need support or practice in every one of these areas, making the initial NHDA an important tool in tweaking what kinds of experiences are planned for the Nurture Nook in various sessions.

If the therapist is trained in Eye Movement Desensitization and Reprocessing (EMDR) therapy (Shapiro, 2017), the Nurture Nook is a perfect place to further install or enhance resources related to the attachment figure (Gomez, 2012). At first, some families may find the intimacy of a Nurture Nook threatening and will need to have *in vivo* experiences of resting together with the support of a therapist before they are able to do so at home. Many of the adopted children whom we see at Nurture House began life in institutional settings. In these settings, nurturing interaction with an adult is a limited resource. Finding the growing edge of a child's Window of Tolerance requires time and patience. These children often are held much less frequently than children raised by good enough parents in biologically intact families. Moreover, many of these children are brought home after a control foundation (which has as its marker the core belief *I must control everything at all costs or I'll die*) has been firmly established. These children see intimacy as risk and restful reliance on a caregiver as excruciatingly uncomfortable. To this end, some of our early work with adopted children and their parents involves expanding the child's Window of Tolerance for restful contact. What does this look like? It can be as simple as having a parent and child sit in close physical proximity to one another while the parent reads a picture book out loud. To some, this would seem "too simple" to be considered therapeutic, but we see many parents who describe their children as so dysregulated that they "will not sit still" to be read to at home. For the child with a deeply entrenched control foundation, even allowing the parent to read to her may feel like she is giving up some of her power. The dyad may need for these experiences to be supported by the therapist *in vivo* in order for both partners to truly relax into restful interaction and to experience pleasurable feedback from this joint attention task. Once the task is experienced as quieting, pleasurable, and safe, these quiet, connected moments can be further enhanced with EMDR therapy.

I have recently been experiencing this with an adopted boy who used to rage uncontrollably. Ricky, a 6-year-old adopted at 3 days old and diagnosed as mildly autistic, had his first of many sessions with me in his family's car, as he refused to come into the building. We began to titrate doses of storytelling and playful inter-action in the car and eventually we were able to transfer this work into a Nurture Nook within the building. I frequently work with families who are in such distress that it is difficult for them to imagine even reading a book together. To read a book together requires a child to be internally regulated enough to be intellectually curi-ous about the story and physically regulated enough to sit tucked up next to Mom or Dad for a period of time.

When I see children with severe attachment disturbances, this can be impos-sible at first. We move toward doses of facilitated storytime. Often I sit between the parent and child and read the first couple of pages of a book. I have previously placed the EMDR therapy buzzies in the child's socks or pockets and, after reading the first couple of pages, trade places with the parent. I facilitate the snuggling up of parent and child and they read together. The feeling of connection, the child's enjoyment of the story, and the trust in the parent that is required to allow her to tell the story up close and personal are further developed with slow short sets of bilateral stimulation (BLS).

The photograph in Figure 6.3 was taken during a session in which this mother and son were both snuggled under the blanket in a posture of relational rest. Ricky has the buzzies in his hands, which was his preferred method of bilateral stimulation, and Mom was reading. This was the first day that the dyad was able to complete a book together, which the therapist had seen as questionable in the beginning. It is worth noting that this was the fifth successful *in vivo* experience in which the mom had read to her child. The first few books were engaging, lighthearted books with pictures that were likely to capture the young boy's attention, mitigating the approach to restful relationship with adventure and developmentally appropriate excitement. We had been titrating the amount of time reading and the difficulty of the content over the course of these sessions. Today's story was about a prickly porcupine who had been adopted. Both parent and child seemed pleased with themselves as Mom completed the story with the words *The End*. What might look like, to an outsider, a normal rhythm of parent–child interaction, was, to all three of us, a major movement toward healing and trust.

Parents will also say that they are bewildered by how much connected time, energy, encouragement, or nurture they can pour into their child—potentially spending the whole day just focused on what the child would like to do next, only to have the child return 2 hours later and say that she "never" gets time with her parent, or she "never" is able to watch what she wants. This experience has been so pervasive for our families that we have created a graphic just to normalize this experience. We call it the "Compromised Container" (see Figure 6.4). If we return to the concepts regarding brain development and our neurophysiological systems discussed in Chapter 2, we remember that when a brain has had the scaffolding it's needed in the reptilian brain to maintain regulation even in the face of stress, then the limbic brain has had the scaffolding it's needed to maintain a sense of connection even in the face of stress. And as a result, the thinking brain can remember good, connected moments of time when the child must do hard or boring things,

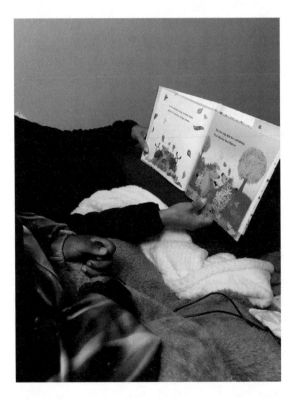

FIGURE 6.3. Absorbing Rest and Snuggles with EMDR.

A COMPROMISED CONTAINER

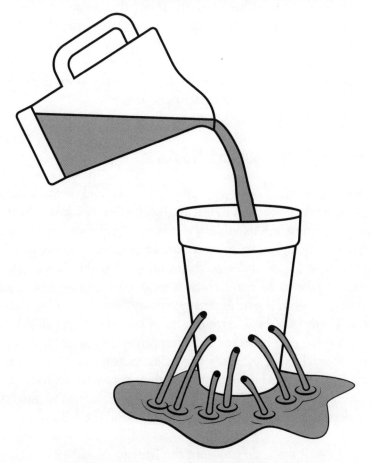

FIGURE 6.4. A Compromised Container.

like homework or getting ready for bed. Most of our clients have injuries to their developing brain, either from *in utero* threats, neglect, maltreatment, or genetic predispositions to dysregulation. For these brains, the moment of pleasure may only be held for that moment. Whereas with typically developing children, a dose of fun and connected time a couple of times a week may sustain them through the monotonous routines of school, children with trauma in their backgrounds often live in the moment, unable to rehearse and revisit other pleasurable moments. All of those good feelings they may have had disappear in the moment that stress is reintroduced. I often compare the parent's experience of these children as similar to the Styrofoam cup that has holes poked in it. The parent keeps pouring in nurture and fun while helping the child build healthy life skills. But, it's as if what the mother or father is pouring in just runs right out again. The child isn't able to keep hold of the things that have been poured in. We offer the parents a copy of the "Compromised Container" handout and ask them to identify the things that they are intentionally pouring into the child in their care that the child isn't able to hold onto. We then discuss the importance of the daily dose of these experiences for their children and begin designing a home Nurture Nook for these families.

Creating Home-Based Nurture Nooks

Once the parent–child dyad or larger family system has had several successful, supported experiences of connection in one of the Nurture Nooks at Nurture House, then we begin to brainstorm together about how to give them this kind of experience at home. The therapist offers the worksheet pictured in Figure 6.5. This handout is meant to help the dyad design their at-home Nurture Nook. This Nurture Nook has several proscribed parameters: It must offer snuggle space, soft fabrics, and plush materials (even if part of our therapeutic work is making these together in the office). There must be a certain level of boundaried smallness (Goodyear-Brown, 2019), a space that helps the child feel protected and calm.

One of the pitfalls that even seasoned therapists cannot avoid is to offer the nugget of an idea to parents for application in their home environment, but without enough structure for them to successfully implement it through scaffolding. To this end, this handout is meant to provide structure around the following decisions:

1. Where in your home do you want the Nurture Nook?
2. How will the boundaries of the space be defined?
3. What sensory experiences do you want to support in this space (e.g., textures of fabrics, lighting, smells, sounds)?
4. Which relational patterns/experiences do you want to re-create in the Nurture Nook?

Let's take a look at these one at a time. Asking the parent and child to decide on a location for the Nurture Nook will help the dyad troubleshoot potential issues that might come up in the transfer of interactions to the home setting. A Nurture Nook may be most helpful if it is not in the corner of a busy room, like the living room, bonus room, or kitchen. It should also be clearly distinct from any space that a family may use for a time-out, or to calm down or reflect on something. Those spaces are meant to de-stimulate the environment for a child, encourage him to regulate physically and potentially think about his behavior—meaning they may be used for a time-out or time-in by families, with either occurring in the wake of some negative interaction, big behaviors, or displays of big feelings by the client.

DESIGNING YOUR NURTURE NOOK

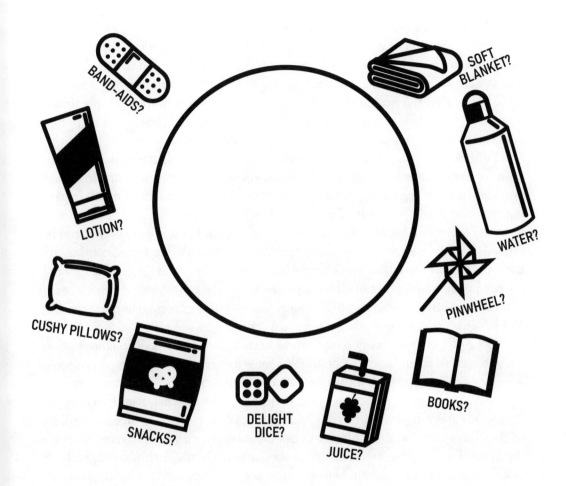

CIRCLE THE ITEMS YOU NEED IN YOUR NURTURE NOOK.

Draw any other items that you might need to include.

FIGURE 6.5. Designing a Nurture Nook.

The Nurture Nook, on the other hand, is a purely pleasurable place of connection between parent and child. It is likely to become an anticipated space of intimacy and relational fun and should not be confused with consequences or discipline of any kind.

The second question, how will the boundaries be defined, helps parents understand more about giving visual indicators to children. A specific blanket may be laid down to create boundaries for the space. A rounded cushion may be used, or a bed in a spare bedroom, or if an environment with more containment is needed, a play-tent or even a huggle pod can be used. Many children are naturally drawn to creating forts, and a semipermanent fort made from old sheets and chip clips attached to furniture pieces can also become a Nurture Nook.

Because the sensory needs of children differ, but are intimately tied to their sense of connection with the world around them, knowing which materials will provide the most regulating input for these Nurture Nook times is worth exploring with the dyad. Supersoft fabrics? Rough natural-fiber materials? Silky smooth textures? Many children are now enjoying those sequin-covered pillows that can be pushed one way or another to create designs, as they provide deep sensory input. As the child strokes the pillow, the kinesthetic regulation provided serves as an anchor for her limbic brain to receive messages of love, and her thinking brain to begin making connections between nurture and identity—thoughts such as I am *delightful* and I am *worthy of nurture* are given room to grow.

Once these logistical questions have been answered, a deeper conversation about which relational patterns or attachment-enhancing experiences can be reenacted at home may be had. If the clinician has been using Theraplay interventions, the dyad might decide that an at-home boo-boo routine is what is most needed, so Band-Aids and lotion will be very important. Specific books may need to be kept in the Nurture Nook, as children will ask for them over and over again. Tools for direct need meeting, such as favorite snacks, a water bottle with a strong suck, or pieces of gum, may be identified as items to keep on hand. When helping parents design Nurture Nooks at home, we ask that parents leave their phones on silent mode somewhere outside of the Nurture Nook and, unless the child has a sensory need that is met by keeping their shoes on, that both parent and child take off their shoes before entering the Nurture Nook.

Parents appreciate the practical support around designing their Nurture Nooks. If mirroring activities (for enhancement of attunement between the dyad) are important, then making sure musical instruments are included in their Nurture Nook could be important. The therapist first leads parent and child in rhythm games in the playroom, offering each a drum or a set of maracas, having the child create a rhythm and asking the mother to match it. Taking turns leading and following in the music making. Other families may need more of a focus on sensory regulation, in which case a weighted blanket or a weighted lap pad, as well as some Chewelry, might have to be incorporated into the Nurture Nook. Parents with lots of financial resources may be able to just run right out, buy their own papasan cushion, and many brand-new books or Band-Aids for use in the Nurture Nook. However, families with very few financial resources can make many of the items that might be needed in a Nurture Nook during the course of therapy. For example, maracas can be made by decorating the cardboard cores of two rolls of toilet paper, then putting some dried beans or rice inside, and covering their ends with Press 'n Seal. These maracas can be created in the playroom, the therapist can ask the dyad to play some games with them in session, and then they can be taken home for continued play.

Some families enjoy making a Nurture Nook bag or basket while in the playroom that can hold all the supplies they need for their Nurture Nook time at home. Offering a bin full of felt pieces, scraps of cloth, ribbons, as well as needle, thread, and a hot glue gun, might be all a parent and child need to begin developing their Nurture Nook bag together. Dyads can become super creative with this activity.

Children who come from institutional settings are often lacking in an internalized template for how we take care of one another. For the most part, tiny humans come into the world with relational capacity: In other words, they have all the ingredients they need to develop empathy and deep care in relationship to others. If they have a good enough caregiver—defined as someone who meets needs thousands and thousands of times in the first year of life, delights in the child at least some of the time, and opens and closes circles of communication regularly— that child lays down the neural scaffolding that implicitly equips him or her to receive care later in life and to give care to others. What we talk about as "natural" nurturing capacities are deeply tied to the kinds of care we received early in life. When clinicians are working with children who grew up in environments devoid of nurturing care, who were neglected or maltreated, these children may not have a template, a mental schema, for what good enough caregiving involves. For these reasons, hurt children may perceive direct caregiving, including nurturing touch, tone, and caretaking, to be uncomfortable, intrusive, or even scary. Taking care of hurts can extend to "loveys" or transitional objects that are in need of some repair. Some of the children whom we see will not be able to receive nurture directly from their own parent when they enter treatment, but may choose other vulnerable creatures in need of care and then carefully watch how the caregiver and/or the therapist takes care of them. Parents sometimes need coaching in understanding the process of vicariously nurturing objects in the Nurture Nook as a way to build safety with their child and to fill their trust tank. Parents may even need to be taught how to speak directly to a stuffed animal/miniature/lovey in the same loving tones and with the same level of nurture that they would like to offer directly to their guarded child. Some parents have playful tendencies or pretend abilities already; others are excruciatingly uncomfortable with pretend play, modulating their voices, the taking on of characters, and the like. These parents may need collateral sessions with you to role-play scenarios and grow their play abilities prior to having sessions with the child who may require them to speak to a lovey or a puppet.

In TraumaPlay, we call it Nurture by Proxy. Jimmy, an 8-year-old boy adopted in the United States, has been unable to receive nurture directly from his mom for years. Several sessions were spent using the sand tray as a focal point for all three of us. We handpicked miniatures to narrate the kinds of early care that babies need—choosing miniature foods to represent meals, soft pieces of fabric to represent loveys, and so on. Jimmy began to pipe up. At first, Mom and I would tell these stories to each other, asking questions, just to one another, about what babies need. Then we moved to wondering out loud what would happen if a baby didn't get what he needed? After several of these sessions, I began to make connections with the client's early life . . . wondering how Mom would attempt to soothe him. Jimmy interjected, "She got me lovey!" Mom smiled broadly and told the story of how he got it on his first birthday. Eventually, a blankie was also identified, and the client talked about how the lovey was "broken" and the blankie had been torn. I asked if Mom could bring in the broken lovey and the torn blankie, along with some needle and thread, for the next session. Jimmy seemed really excited about this idea, and at the next session they brought in a bag full of broken toys that needed to be stitched up or patched. I first explained that since needles can hurt, Jimmy would need his Safe Boss to help him thread the needle and use it. Jimmy, who had been aggressive many times with sharp objects, used incredible care in handling the needle. It made me think of the Spider-Man mantra "With great power comes great responsibility." Jimmy and his mom began with the loveys he had brought from home. They told stories about where the loveys had come from as they fixed them. They mended the loveys by connecting one side of the torn fabric (out of which stuffing was falling) to the other side of the torn fabric. As loop after loop of string was sewn through the two sides, pulling them closer and closer together, a parallel process was happening inside of Jimmy. He began allowing himself to move closer and closer to mom, both emotionally and in terms of allowing her to help bring coherence to his story. It was a powerful piece of work. After they were finished, Jimmy said, "I saw that one of your pillows has a hole in it. Would you like us to sew it?" I accepted the offer with great delight, and Jimmy and his mom got to work finding some grey thread and cooperatively sewing the Nurture Nook pillow (see Figure 6.6). Jimmy was experiencing a competency surge that was only possible for him in this way as he risked allowing his Safe Boss to help him. He felt so connected to her, he used the "we" to offer that they fix my pillow together.

Many children who come from hard places have not had the experience of being put to bed in a loving way. This understanding that some children can only receive nurture vicariously to start informs one of my prompts in the play therapy space. I will often offer baby dolls, pillows, and blankets and help parents enact putting the babies to bed while the child watches (see Figure 6.7). After a child has watched mom and/or me take care of the baby doll lovingly, the child can risk asking for nurture more directly.

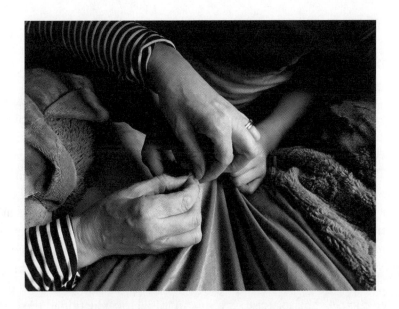

FIGURE 6.6. Nurturing Repair in the Nook.

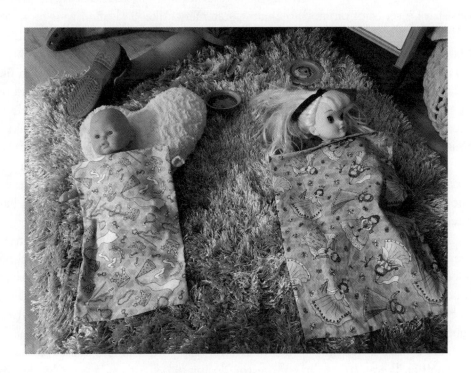

FIGURE 6.7. Vicarious Nurture.

Love Languages and Delighting-In Dice

One of the games that we play in the Nurture Nook is a dice game in which various forms of giving and receiving love are practiced. As with most new activities that involve the child, we begin by having the parent work with us to understand the how and why of the activity. Some parents will come to therapy having already read about the "Love Languages." These parents will be able to identify their own primary Love Language and also their child's right away. Other parents will need time to explore their own love wiring as well as their children's. The Love Languages were identified by Gary Chapman (1995). He posits that there are five main ways that we give and receive love: quality time, words of affirmation, physical touch, acts of service, and gifts. We have large six-sided, dry-erase cubes that we keep for this game. We write one Love Language on each side as we describe each (the sixth side is a free choice). This exercise serves as an initial introduction to the categories. When such content is new to families, we take some time playfully completing the Love Languages profile (which can be found at *5lovelanguages.com*). The profile consists of a series of prompts, including statements like "I cleaned your room for you," "Give me a kiss," "You are an awesome kid!," "Let's play a game together," "Look under your bed for a special surprise!" We print out a copy of all the prompts and cut them up so that each prompt is about the size of a fortune that you would find stuffed in a fortune cookie. The parent and child take turns picking out one paper prompt at a time and reading it out loud. As parent and child become sleuths together, they discover which kind of prompt the child chooses most often. Once family members have identified their primary Love Language, the dry-erase die is brought back out as well as smaller, foam dice—enough for each person in the session to have one. Each person gets a copy of Figure 6.8 and, after filling in their primary Love Language, identifies six personalized ways in which they would like to receive love.

If the child's Love Language is physical touch, his six behavioral expressions of love might read: hugs, high fives, snuggle, fist bumps, back rubs, thumb wrestling. Once these have been encoded on the handout, the therapist leads family members through the creation of their own delighting-in die, personalized with each of these six behavioral expressions. Examples of several Delighting-In Dice are shown in Figure 6.9.

As we work to enhance attachments and help parents and children attune to one another, therapists can maximize the dosing of delight when we help identify the best ways for children to absorb nurture. Giving and receiving love can be more complicated than families may think. Let's say a parent feels loved when she receives physical touch. This parent is likely to give love to her children in the same way that she receives it herself. So, she may hug her children often, attempt to snuggle up really close to read books, or attempt to hold her son's hand as they are walking through the mall. This will work wonderfully to build a connection if the

WORKSHEET FOR DELIGHTING-IN DICE

Every person has a primary way in which
they give and receive love. Using the dice below,
identify your primary portal for receiving delight.

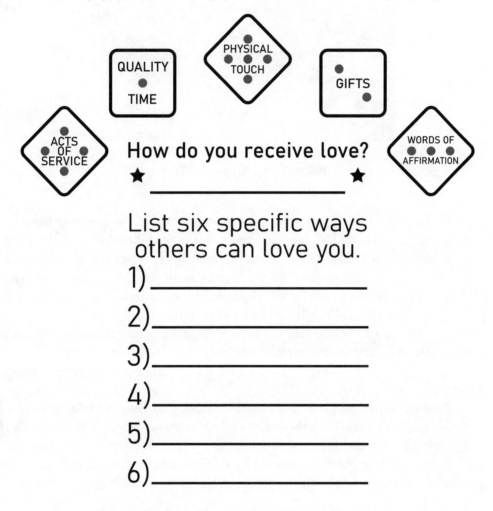

FIGURE 6.8. Delighting-In Dice Worksheet.

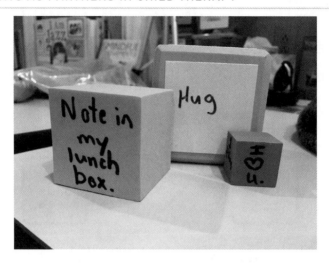

FIGURE 6.9. Personalized Dice.

child is also wired to receive love through physical touch. However, if the child is actually wired to receive love mostly through words of affirmation, that child may not get his love tank filled by his mom. An even worse mismatch would occur if the child also had some sensory differences that made touch uncomfortable. This child could experience Mom's "love" as painful. In yet another scenario, the mom who gives lots of physical touch may have a latency-age child who has decided he really doesn't want to be touched in public. Any of these mismatches could cause further disconnection in the attachment relationship—thus, the importance of helping parents and children practice meeting each other's needs in their own Love Language.

Once all participants have completed Delighting-In Dice, we take turns playing with each die, practicing the behavioral expressions within session. We then assign the parent and child to carve out 5 minutes of delighting-in time using the dice in their Nurture Nook at home each day. This practice both in and out of session helps parents and children to strengthen their love connections.

Delighting-In Stories

Another standard activity that we include in our Nurture Nook time with families is Delighting-In Stories. These serve three purposes: (1) The child feels good as she hears the parent telling a story about her delightfulness. (2) The parent gets practice in storytelling while using positive content to prepare for later storytelling that may involve bringing coherence to more difficult content. (3) A culture of storytelling is established within the family, and the parent is promoted as a Storykeeper for the child. A script for helping parents create Delighting-In Stories is presented in Figure 6.10.

Delighting-In Story Starters

During each session, we will have you tell a story in which you get to do one of the following:

1) Celebrate a new competency that your child has developed or an achievement. Examples include:
   a. Learning to ride a bike
   b. Reading for 20 minutes out loud
   c. Making their own breakfast or lunch

2) Rehearse a moment of humor or delight from the week. Examples include:
   a. A time that they told a joke
   b. That night when they did a silly dance before bed
   c. The time you played three rounds of thumb wars and they won every time

3) Give the details of a prosocial choice or choice to use self-control that was clearly hard for them, but they did it anyway. Examples include:
   a. The time that they came and told you when their sister was bothering them
   b. When they sat with you at dinner for a long time and then politely asked to be excused
   c. When they could have taken the last cookie, but instead shared it with their brother

4) Describe, in detail, a caretaking moment. Examples include:
   a. A time when they had a boo-boo and came to you to take care of it
   b. A time when you both took care of a pet together
   c. A time when you made food that they liked and they ate it all up

5) Any time when they used their voice to ask for what they needed.

Story starters are below:

1) When you were a baby, I used to snuggle you and you would . . .

2) I need to brag on Johnny . . . he has been working so hard on . . . and just this week . . .

3) We had a super silly moment together earlier this week when Johnny . . .

4) Johnny and I baked cookies together . . . I broke the eggs and he stirred in the flour . . .

5) Earlier this week Johnny really needed _____ and I wasn't understanding yet, and he was able to use his good words to ask for what he needed . . .

FIGURE 6.10. Delighting-In Story Starters.

Humbugs

Another intervention that is easily completed in the Nurture Nook helps to amplify the potential for parent and child to participate in mindfulness practice together. This lovely intervention combines breath work and shared humming (which stimulate the vagus nerve and invite more social connectedness between parents and children). Eleah Hyatt, a talented play therapist and part of our team at Nurture House, designed this intervention called "Humbugs." Treatment goals include the following:

1. To introduce mindfulness and the benefits of being able to calm oneself through vagal nerve stimulation
2. To teach self-regulation through a form of vagal nerve stimulation
3. To help the parent–child dyad gain an awareness of ways to achieve a state of focused relaxation and calming through the activation of the vagal nerve
4. To increase self-empowerment and feelings of control over one's mind and body
5. To provide an opportunity for co-regulation between client and a safe adult who can join the client in this self-regulation activity
6. To help strengthen clients' understanding and appreciation for the mind–body connection

The procedures are as follows:

Learning and using proper breathing techniques is one of the most beneficial things that can be done for both short- and long-term physical and emotional health. Abdominal breathing helps to relax the nervous system, reduces stress and tension, lowers blood pressure, and calms the mind. Practicing abdominal breathing also massages and tones the internal organs, particularly the digestive organs.

The means by which controlled breathing triggers the parasympathetic nervous system is linked to stimulation of the vagus nerve—a nerve running from the base of the brain to the abdomen and responsible for mediating nervous system responses and lowering the heart rate, among other functions.

The vagus nerve releases a neurotransmitter called acetylcholine that catalyzes increased focus and calmness. A direct benefit of more acetylcholine is a decrease in feelings of anxiety. Stimulating the vagus nerve may also play a role in treating depression, even in people who are resistant to anti-depressant medications. There are many ways to stimulate vagal nerve activity and increase heart rate variability. Some of them include singing, humming, mantra chanting, hymn singing, upbeat energetic singing, and "Om" chanting. Humbugs is a creative activity that helps kids connect a concrete object to mindfulness and self-regulating skills they've learned and further serves as a visual reminder that they can access outside of session at home or school.

This activity begins by providing the client with a developmentally appropriate

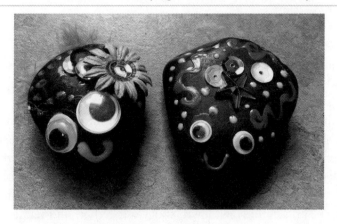

FIGURE 6.11. Humbugs.

rationale for self-regulation and mindfulness skills. The therapist may also provide some psychoeducation around the mind–body connection and its role in one's overall well-being and health.

Start by selecting rocks to use for creating the Humbugs. Rocks may be found outside during a mindfulness walk with the client, if you are able to do this at your practice location. Otherwise, rocks may be purchased at local craft or dollar stores. Rocks should be small enough to fit in a pant, coat, or backpack pocket and the client should be given two rocks, one for each hand. Provide the client with various craft materials of different colors and textures that she can use to create her Humbugs. Encourage the client to mindfully select craft items and identify as many of the five senses as possible in her selection. Once the Humbugs are complete and dried, brainstorm with the client on situations in which she may need to calm and regulate herself at home or school. Apply the knowledge she has already learned about the vagal nerve and the ways in which its activation through humming or Om-ing can help calm the mind and body. Invite the client to gently squeeze her Humbug in each hand as she focuses on humming or Om-ing together with you or a safe caregiver or parent. The client may also practice grounding herself by visually noticing the colors and textures of the Humbug she's created. After a few rounds of humming or Om-ing, process the mind–body impact of this activity together. Completed Humbugs are shown in Figure 6.11.

Rehearsal Roses

I love it when our clients teach us things. Recently, I was facilitating attachment-enhancement work with an adopted child and his mother. We had settled into a Nurture Nook, and I had brought along a hard surface and some sculpting clay, thinking that I might invite them to create something together in the clay. I had no real plan in mind, which is sometimes when the magic happens. The son—we'll call him Daniel—had a rough day at school and had not really shaken it off by the time he arrived at the Nurture Nook. He was stony with silence and unwilling to make eye contact. Thinking through the play therapist's palette (Goodyear-Brown, 2019), I asked myself what he might need to help him get unstuck. Kinesthetic involvement is often the most powerful way to begin gently shaking a child out of a freeze/withdrawal response, so I invited Mom to narrate the frustrating events of the day as she might if she had been in his shoes that day. While she narrated, I pulled out one chunk of clay and put it in front of Mom, and then pulled out a second chunk of clay and put it in front of Daniel (which he immediately tossed to the side); I next pulled off a chunk for myself. I believe that magic can occur when we help a parent and child slow down, snuggle together, and relate to each other in a relaxed and contained environment. Adding the offered options of kinesthetic involvement in the manipulation of the clay and the clay as a focal point for visual attention decreases the sense of threat that a fear-based brain might otherwise find alarming.

Mom started pulling off small balls of clay and flattening them. She said that she was making something and winked at Daniel. I watched as she rolled out a ball into a quarter-sized, flat circle of clay. She did that three more times and then began to overlay one circle on top of the other. Daniel reached out and said, "You're doing it wrong!" and was about to move one of her pieces when I reminded him that he had clay of his own, so he would need to ask Mom if he could change what she was making. He sighed, rolled his eyes, and then reached out and grabbed the piece of clay he had tossed aside. I said that I wasn't sure what they were making but couldn't wait to see. We talked more about the hard day while Daniel and his mother continued pulling off small balls of clay, flattening them into circles and laying them one on top of the other in long chains. After they had each made 8 to 10 circles, Mom smiled at me and said, "Wait for it." She and Daniel made eye contact, and he sort of smiled; then starting at one end of their chains, they rolled up the clay. When they were done rolling, they held up the clay: What had been created was a beautiful rose before its petals have unfurled. They were so cool.

I exclaimed, "Wow! Your flowers are amazing . . . and watching the process had me thinking this could be a good intervention for helping parents and kids celebrate each other. Would you be willing to help me design it?" Daniel was eager to show me how to make the circles and delighted in telling me when I had made one too small or too large. I introduced other colors of clay, and I asked each of them to make a rose for the other. Each petal represented something that each appreciated about the other. Daniel had a hard time at first, but I helped and he ended up creating circles while saying things such as "I like the way you get me Subway sandwiches" or "Thanks for buying me a Fortnite skin this week." This client's MO is to pretend he hates being nice or seen as kind, while secretly enjoying both being positively talked about and complimenting others. Each of them got to take home their roses, which we decided to call Rehearsal Roses, as they encouraged the out loud rehearsal of positive aspects of their relationship (see Figure 6.12).

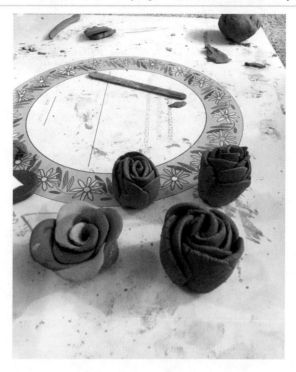

FIGURE 6.12. Rehearsal Roses.

Penguin Praises

I am not a fan of put-on praise, the Pollyanna praise that a teacher might give to two or three children—"Thank you for sitting in your seat, thank you for sitting in your seat . . ."—while she is really trying to just get the one child who won't sit down to do so. However, I am a big fan of expressing genuine appreciation and thanks for the kindnesses that we do for one another, especially in family systems that may need the practice. Recently, on a trip through China, I found a beautiful pair of penguins (see Figure 6.13). I was drawn to them because they clearly stick together with one another, but it took some exploration to figure out that they are hollow and their backs open up, with each penguin providing some storage space (see Figure 6.14). I was charmed by the pair and immediately began using them in the Nurture Nook as part of a beginning ritual, inviting both parent and child to quiet themselves for a moment, reflect on the week, and identify one service that the other provided to them. The child's examples might include mommy reading her a story, daddy cutting her hotdog into pieces, and mommy taking her to school. The parent's examples might include a son taking out the trash, a daughter making her mom a cup of tea, or both children cleaning up after dinner. I provide pads of small sticky notes and have each participant write down one thing they appreciate about the other from the current week. I encourage the child and parent to fold up the tiny pieces of paper even tinier and put them in the penguins' backs. We set

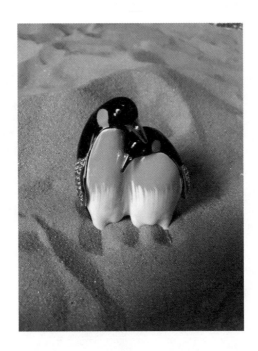

FIGURE 6.13. Penguins Sticking Together.

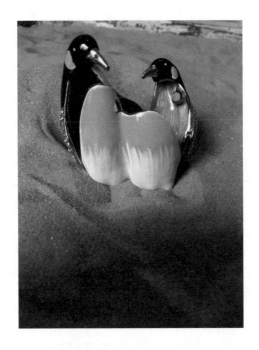

FIGURE 6.14. Open Penguins.

these figurines off to the side, anticipating reading the appreciations later on in session. In some families, this has become a part of the beginning and closing rituals that must not be missed.

All of the therapeutic interventions offered thus far for enhancing delighting-in experiences for parents and children have been activities that can be completed in the Nurture Nook. There are a couple of other intervention offerings that our families love, but that require more physical space. The first of these is Airplane Love Notes. We believe deeply in the power of gratitude and appreciation. This can be made more fun when parents and children write down their appreciations and send them in paper airplane form to one another. Our supervision team recently completed this activity with one another. Each person was given a brightly colored piece of paper and asked to think of something they appreciate about someone else on our team; then on the count of 3, we sent our airplanes zooming around the room. Having the parent and child each pick a piece of paper, create an airplane, and then zoom them down the hallway or move into the backyard outside space to race the airplanes are also fun activities. Figure 6.15 is a handout that outlines the steps for how to make a paper airplane, if, like me, the parent or child in your care has never been taught this skill.

Beautiful Hand Creations

Beautiful Hands, a stunning book created by Kathryn Otoshi and Bret Baumgarten (2015), shows page after page of ways that our hands, fingers, and fingerprints can be used to create flowers, birds, butterflies, ladybugs, and even dragons. One of my favorite dyadic works is a butterfly made by arranging two splayed handprints of the parent and two handprints of the child to represent the wings of the butterfly. Then an individual finger can make up the middle of the body or this can be drawn in, and a thumbprint becomes the head of the butterfly (see Figure 6.16). Many times, children are unwilling to receive nurturing touch if it is too overtly offered, but the touch necessitated by painting each other's hands as a step toward the larger goal of creating a work of art together normally mitigates the approach by even our most touch-aversive clients to this activity. Many of our parents are also hungry to provide this direct nurturing to their child, and very few words are needed to create something that is unique to the family system.

We start by reading the book together in the Nurture Nook. The therapist facilitates a conversation in which a parent and child together choose the kind of design they want to make. Since many of the children we see have short attention spans, it is helpful to have prepared the space where you are going to do this activity in advance, providing the paints, paper, paintbrushes, and a water source for handwashing afterward. The parent asks the child what colors he would like on his hand, modeling choice-giving and following the child's lead. The parent gently holds the child's hand underneath for support while painting his fingers.

PAPER AIRPLANE LOVE NOTES

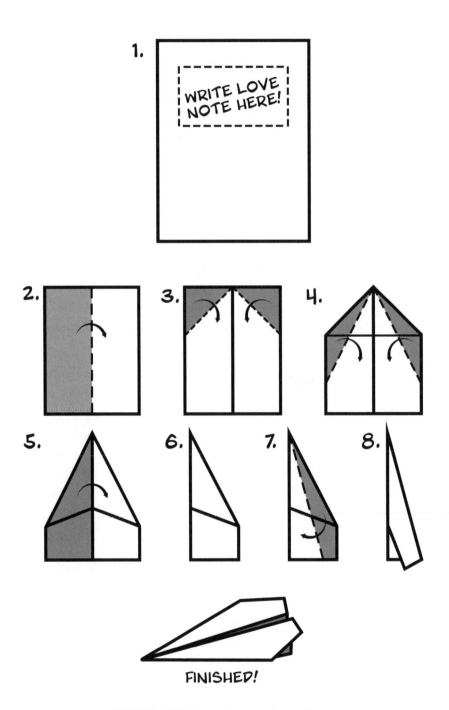

FIGURE 6.15. Paper Airplane Love Notes.

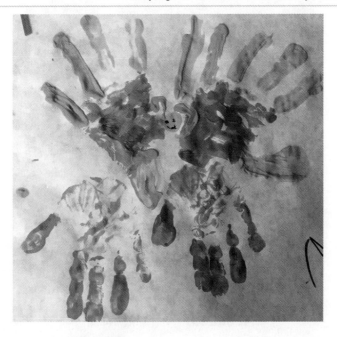

FIGURE 6.16. Creating Hope Together.

Both parent and child usually have their eyes focused on the child's hand as it is being painted, which mitigates the level of intimacy in the activity (see Figure 6.17). Shown here is a beautiful hand creation made by a whole family: It became a bird (see Figure 6.18). Many of our families take home their creations and frame them.

Funsequences

Parents are raising children in a sea of cultural messages about self, consumerism, and entertainment. In the midst of this culture, most parents work valiantly to instill a set of values in their children that embrace the power of hard work, combat the pull of procrastination, and highlight the importance of being part of a team and of everyone pitching in. Parents have often absorbed the basics of rewards and consequences and are good at communicating these to their children. The reward of studying for your test is that you receive an A, which sets you up for getting into a good college and eventually having a meaningful career. The consequence of not studying is that you fail the test, get low grades, and narrow the scope of colleges to which you will be accepted, thereby narrowing your career choices as well. In the daily rhythms of family life, parents frequently provide additional consequences when family responsibilities are not met. If you don't do the dishes, then you don't get your screen time after dinner. In families with high-achieving members, the studying gets completed and the dishes get washed. Everyone performs at a high level, and there is general family harmony . . . which is not the same as family fun.

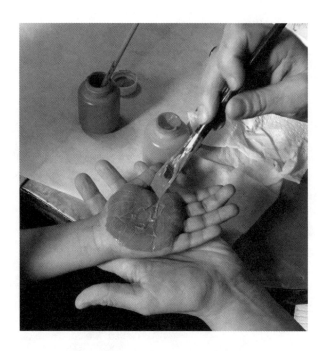

FIGURE 6.17. Nurturing Touch.

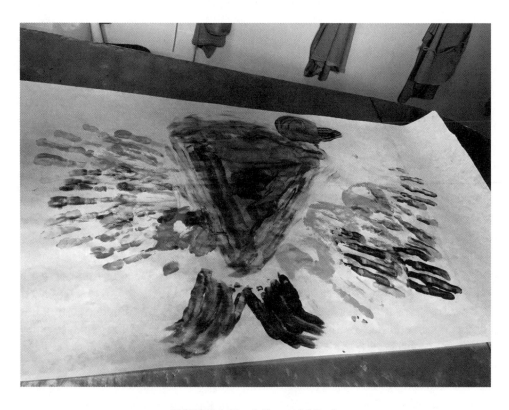

FIGURE 6.18. A Beautiful Bird.

If we are going to provide consequences within a family when chores are not done, can't we also provide Funsequences for the whole family when everyone has done the hard things that need doing? A Funsequence is an activity that the family engages in together, particularly after all have done the hard things. The hard thing looks different for children of different ages. Let's say the children are 3, 9, and 12. The 12-year-old may have the job of reading two chapters of a book: for him, a hard thing. The 9-year-old may have the job of falling into the pattern of remembering to get his planner signed each night and to make his lunch for the next day. The 3-year-old may have the job of sitting on the potty multiple times a day while potty training. All the children have jobs—hard things that need doing. Parents who value the hard work of their children and celebrate the hard work of all are more likely to develop a healthy balance of work and play than those who do not.

One recent week in our family, my oldest son Sam, who is a high-school senior, had the first draft of his thesis due; my daughter Madison, who is a freshman in high school, had to memorize and recite an ancient Greek poem; and my youngest son Nicholas, who is a fourth grader, had to write, memorize, and recite a speech to the entire grammar school. I had 2 days of traveling to speak to a couple of hundred people on the TraumaPlay model, 10 pages to write for the next book, and many clients/supervisees to care for. My travel meant that my husband had to navigate his work schedule while taking up the slack for getting the children everywhere they needed to go. The oldest two help with babysitting our youngest, so extra responsibilities went along with that while I was out of town. Large responsibilities, deadlines, and hard things for each of us. There would be real-life consequences for each of us if we individually dropped the ball, and real-life consequences for us as a family unit if we individually or collectively dropped the ball. So, why shouldn't there also be real-life Funsequences for us as a family when we fulfill our obligations?

We call these Family Funsequences and model them after the Disney Song Challenge board game we discovered on a family outing to a local coffee shop. Our family keeps Sundays as sacrosanct family time, and we maintain a running list of activities that we do together. The activities themselves are fun, but doing them together keeps a focus on the family unit as a place where fun is created. Families run at an incredibly intense pace, and carving out time for Family Funsequences can reinforce the family's sense that families that play together stay together. The challenge can be finding activities that are fun for all family members. To this extent, having the clinician facilitate conversation around Funsequences while guiding clients in identifying the first Funsequence offered by each family member, using photocopies of the tickets reproduced in Figure 6.19, can set the family up for success.

FUNSEQUENCES

FAMILY FUNSEQUENCE

This ticket entitles the _____ family
to one _____ .

Compliments of _____
<small>(Insert family member name here.)</small>

FAMILY FUNSEQUENCE

This ticket entitles the _____ family
to one _____ .

Compliments of _____
<small>(Insert family member name here.)</small>

FAMILY FUNSEQUENCE

This ticket entitles the _____ family
to one _____ .

Compliments of _____
<small>(Insert family member name here.)</small>

This tool is meant to help focus families on cooperation and to help them celebrate
cooperative success together. Invite your children to a family meeting.
Make a list of the kinds of behaviors/achievements/communication patterns that can help
the family earn Funsequences. Invite all family members to add to the list of potential Funsequences.
Some examples follow: one afternoon picnic by the lake, 1 hour of board game play,
one baking project, one family walk in the woods.

FIGURE 6.19. Funsequences.

CHAPTER 7

Helping Parents Train the Triune Brain

We introduced a graphic representation of the triune brain in Chapter 2. There, we unpacked an understanding of bottom-up brain development as a way to set the stage for where parents should be setting the bar (Rothschild, 2000). In this chapter, we will introduce strategies to help parents support all three parts of the triune brain as much as possible. To this end, parents must know which part of the brain they are parenting at any given time. If the child is having a meltdown, is it because his reptilian brain stem is screaming at the child that he needs to eat or sleep, or snuggle? Is the meltdown due to the child's feelings of hurt, and connecting with the parent over this big emotion would be most helpful? Or, is the upset the result of a cognitive distortion that the child believes is true, and the most helpful parenting strategy would be to confront the distortion? Training parents to take a quick scan of the needs of their child can look as simple as asking the following: What is the need underlying the behavior? Is this a regulation issue? Is this a connection issue? Or, is this a thinking brain issue? The parent may get the answer wrong, but at least training the parent to ask this series of questions can equip him or her to hit the mark more often.

Sensory Processing Issues

Sensory processing issues are one of the more insidious causes of division between parents and children by the time they come to treatment. Lots of parents will seek out a mental health solution for what they perceive as children's big behaviors or overwhelming emotions, when an evaluation by an occupational therapist may be what is most needed. In fact, after hearing a family's initial description of their child and asking a few key questions, we will often recommend an occupational therapy evaluation as one of the very next steps for a family. It is a standard part of our intake procedures to ask if a child has any sensory processing issues. Parents will almost always say "no" at first, but as we begin to ask more questions or further explore their previous comments about their child, their eyes may begin to open to sensory issues. Children's neuroception of safety, what we talk to parents about as "felt safety," can be greatly undermined when one or more of their senses is over- or underfunctioning (Kranowitz, 2005; Payne, Levine, & Crane-Godreau, 2015). For example, a mom is potty training her toddler, and the child refuses to sit on the potty. This mom might see her child's avoidance of the potty through the lens of defiance: "He just doesn't want to." The mom might rightly perceive the fear that her child experiences when faced with the task of going to the bathroom, but mis-understand it as a fear of releasing urine into the potty, when it is the sound of the toilet flushing that is overwhelming and scary for the child. This child may be sen-sory defensive when it comes to his auditory encoding. Loud sounds are dysregulat-ing for him, and he will benefit from a parent who can view him through that lens.

We have eight identified sensory systems, and while most of us are only aware of the five senses, understanding more deeply the needs of the physical and sensory self will help us co-regulate the children in our care. We have several swings at Nurture House, and the one that is always used more than I would have imagined is the one pictured in Figure 7.1. Children sit in the middle of this swing and spin and spin . . . and spin and spin . . . far beyond the point when I would have passed out or thrown up. Their proprioceptive and vestibular needs are significantly different from my own, and they are often different than their parent's sensory impressions of the world around them. Learning a child's sensory needs together is part of the work of helping parents become partners in child therapy.

Sensory Savvy

I remember vividly the car ride home from the hospital with the new-born Sam, our now 18-year-old son. We had diligently installed the car seat, even having it checked by a professional service before I went into labor. We had bought special neck pillows that wrapped around the straps of the little baby seat belt. We strapped him in ever so carefully, and his head lolled to the side and down onto his chest in a way that looked incredibly uncomfortable to me. He fell asleep instantly and seemed unphased. I, however, remember thinking in a panic: Isn't there some sort of test we are supposed to take before the hospital can release him to us? I had heard the jokes that you had to have a license to drive a car but that anybody could have a baby, but I hadn't understood the full implication of how underequipped I was until we were driving away from the support of medical professionals. Parenting, at first, is about getting to know the needs of your little one and stepping up to meet them. It becomes clear quickly to most parents when a child is hungry, when she is scared, when she is cold, when she needs to be changed, and parents are deeply gratified

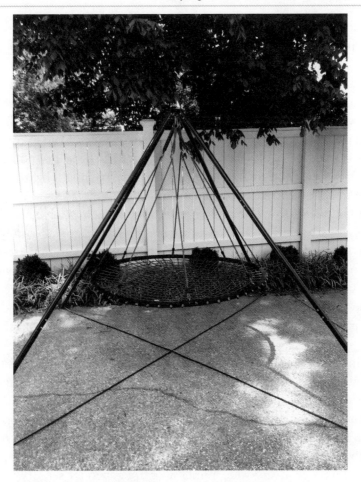

FIGURE 7.1. Spinning Swing.

when something they do to meet a need or to soothe has the response that was intended—the baby is soothed, the baby is warmed, the baby is content and connected. Sensory processing issues throw an enormous wrench into this reciprocity in the relationship between parent and child that is sometimes taken for granted. Children with sensory differences can continue to cry long after they have been fed, or to arch away from a parent who is attempting to cuddle and soothe their infant. If it is true that we don't get a course in basic parenting before we become parents, it is doubly true that we are not given any specialized training about sensory processing differences, yet at least 1 in 20 people is affected by sensory processing disorder (SPD) (Miller, Fuller, & Roetenberg, 2014). The comorbidity rates between SPD and other diagnoses such as attention-deficit/hyperactivity disorder (ADHD), autism, and giftedness are higher than among the average population. Making sensory differences accessible to parents can be challenging, and often mental health professionals are the first to see these children, as the big behaviors that show up as an outgrowth of sensory experiences often push parents to seek counseling. We, as clinicians, are ambassadors of information about the sensory needs of children and frequently the first to refer a child for occupational therapy.

During an intake with a new family, clinicians may ask the question "Does your child have any sensory issues that you are aware of?" If I had a quarter for every time a parent first says "no," but then revises their response to a "yes" when asked additional questions, I would be rich. It is important that child therapists follow up with parents, asking questions such as "Does your child ever complain about the way his clothes feel on his skin?" "Does she restrict herself to just jeans or just dresses?" "Does your child complain about loud noises or bright lights?" "Does your child refuse to eat certain foods, or complain about the textures of certain foods?" "Does your child start to spin out of control when he is in a large busy place (like a mall) or in a very small space?" "Is your child pretty snuggly/physically affectionate or does she not like to be touched?" Having an accurate understanding of a child's sensory needs early in treatment helps us equip parents as co-regulators and children to better understand what their bodies are needing. At Nurture House, we have a wide variety of tools to help client with their proprioceptive and vestibular input. It is particularly rewarding when children begin to tell us what they need to regulate.

The simplest way I have found to talk about sensory differences is to describe the intersection of two processes: how a child takes in information and how she copes with what she takes in. Children take in information related to all their senses all the time. Some children have a low neurological threshold or a narrow Window of Tolerance for sensory input. These children may perceive the beeping of the microwave to be an intolerably loud sound. Other children have a high neurological threshold or a very wide Window of Tolerance for sensory input. These children may be underresponsive to some stimuli. They may not even notice the microwave beeping as they are highly engaged in a task. These two ends of the continuum, low and high, are dotted with a range of sensory experiences and represent how children process information from the environment. The second dimension has to do with how children handle what they take in. We often refer to this as "self-regulation," which is best defined on a behavioral continuum from passive to active. Children who are passive self-regulators will allow uncomfortable sensory experiences to build up and then become reactive. This child may continue to stay on the brightly sunny playground even though the sunlight feels overwhelming.

I am remembering a 6-year-old child, Edward, who was diagnosed with autism and had SPD. He went to a private school that insisted he wear his collar buttoned. He would passively accept this when Mom would button it in the morning, make it through the first 2 hours of the day, and then inevitably experience a meltdown that resulted in him having to go home. Once at home, he took off the shirt and had no more behavioral spikes that day. It took careful data collection and curious exploration to figure out that he was sort of white knuckling it through the first hours of the day, but then his internal resources for regulation were quickly being used up on this tactile coping and the first stressful event of the day (e.g., a spelling test, coming across a word he couldn't read, another child not sharing a ball with him on the playground) required resources he didn't have. Children who are active self-regulators will move themselves away from the bright sunlight in order to cope with the sensory discomfort.

Dunn's model of sensory processing informs my thinking about the importance of understanding the child's sensory profile (Dunn, 2007). The intersection of two continuums—neurological threshold and self-regulation—is posited and results in four distinct presentations for children with SPD. The first is sensory seeking. These children have a high threshold, meaning it takes more of a certain kind of sensory input for them to perceive it, and they are active self-regulators. The second presentation is sensory defensive, or sensory avoidant. These children have a low threshold, perceiving normative amounts of sensory input in one or more categories as too much or too intense, and they are active self-regulators. The third presentation is sensory sensitive. These children have a low threshold for absorbing sensory data and a passive self-regulation pattern. They may stay in uncomfortable environments and eventually seem sad, anxious, or depressed with no precipitating event. The majority of children have the fourth presentation, typically high thresholds and active strategies for self-regulating. We are unlikely to see significant stress or big behaviors from children who fall into this fourth category. The handout in Figure 7.2 is useful to give to parents as clinicians explain the quadrants. What this grid will not show you is the complex presentation that many of our children with equally complex trauma histories have, in which they are sometimes sensory defensive and sometimes sensory seeking. Their sensitivities may vary with the time of day or the season of the year, and are likely to vary from sensory system to sensory system: meaning the children may be sensory seeking in one area (they may want lots of tactile engagement), but sensory defensive in another (they don't like to wear socks with seams or hear people chewing). Figure 7.2 will also prove helpful in explaining these continuums to parents.

My first goal when I see that a parent–child dyad is confused or dismissive about how sensory processing works and why it matters is to expand both the parent and child's knowledge and awareness. We tackle the knowledge piece through playful psychoeducation. I start by asking if they know how many senses we have. Most people know the basic five and can list most of them, but don't know about the other three sensory systems. We have eight sensory systems in all. The five we are most familiar with are as follows:

1. The tactile sense: what we perceive when we touch something
2. The olfactory sense: what we smell
3. The auditory sense: what we hear
4. The gustatory sense: what we taste
5. The visual sense: what we see

NEUROLOGICAL THRESHOLDS FOR SENSORY INPUT

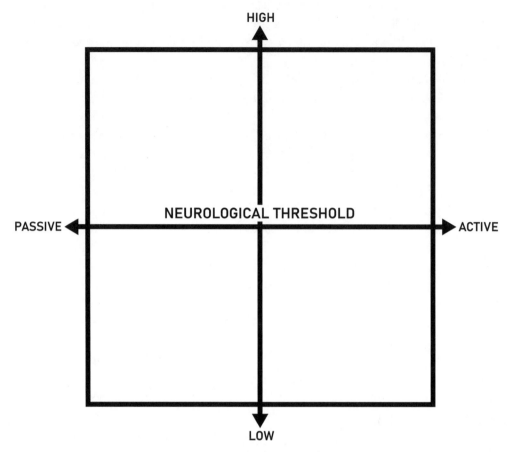

How do you experience the world?
After you've been introduced to the different ways we approach the sensory world, make a dot in the quadrant that best describes you! Add other marks for each of your children.

FIGURE 7.2. Neurological Threshold Handout. Adapted from Dunn (2007).

The sensory systems that will be less familiar to parents and kids are these:

6. Proprioception: the body's ability to sense itself in space
7. Interoception: the body's ability to sense itself from the inside
8. The vestibular sense: largely responsible for balance

The handout in Figure 7.3 is a way to help parents develop a personalized sensory profile for their child, with your help. Using the continuum grid above, parents can reflect on their child's seeking or defensive tendencies in each of the eight senses. Specific strategies for shaping the environment to meet the needs of the minor child can stem from this visual aid.

Your Child's Eight Senses

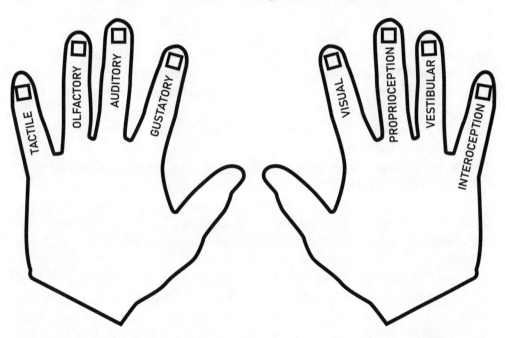

Your child may need more sensory input in some areas and may avoid sensory input in other areas. Using red, blue, and green markers, color in each fingernail as you reflect on your child's sensory systems— red for sensory seeking, blue for sensory defensive, and green for balance.

FIGURE 7.3. Sensory Hands.

The first part of enlisting parents as partners in this work is helping them to understand all eight senses. We put an item to represent each of the senses into a brown paper bag. The child and parent take turns putting their hand in the bag, choosing an object, pulling it out, and then guessing together which sense the object represents. This also becomes a first exposure to honing the tactile sense, as it requires each partner to *feel* what's in the bag. Being able to easily touch things, encode them accurately, and manipulate them kinesthetically seem like basic abilities, so basic that we take them for granted. Yet for some children, the tactile sensations caused by touching an object can be very dysregulating, especially if the object has a texture that is unfamiliar or off-putting to them. Some children can't abide having lotion applied to their bodies. Other children will completely "come apart" if the seams of their socks aren't lined up just right. Those parents who have already embraced their children's unique sensory distress will have made some accommodations. They learn to buy the socks without seams. They learn to give the child a verbal warning before they flush the toilet and perhaps even offer to put their hands over their child's ears. The toughest children are those who are sensory defensive in one or more areas and simultaneously sensory seeking in others. The "Sensory Hands" handout is useful in helping parents think through in which sense areas their child may be sensory seeking, while in others the child may be sensory defensive.

Once we've expanded a family's understanding of the sensory needs of their child, we begin expanding the child's Window of Tolerance for experiencing each of these senses. We often create playful exposure response/prevention hierarchies that move a child from an aversion to the taste or smell of certain foods to an ability to tolerate or even enjoy them. Whenever possible, we integrate play therapy and EMDR therapy in this work, utilizing the Worry Wars Protocol as a way to begin externalizing the anxiety around the sensory experiences (Goodyear-Brown, 2010b, 2011).

We also begin harnessing the sensory experiences that will be supportive to the child as early as possible in this work. We create Sensory Soothing Menus for parents and children alike. It can be very instructive to create one for each family member during a family session. We begin by identifying five parts of a meal, and then pair each part of the meal with one of our five primary senses and identify a pleasurable, calming sensory experience in each of these categories. Examples of a menu cover and a completed menu are given in Figure 7.4 and Figure 7.5, respectively. Figure 7.6 offers a template for creating one with families.

Helping Parents Develop Emotional Granularity and Shared Language with Their Children

Once we have begun addressing the sensory regulation needs of children, as well as meeting their basic needs, we move to helping parents expand their tool kit so

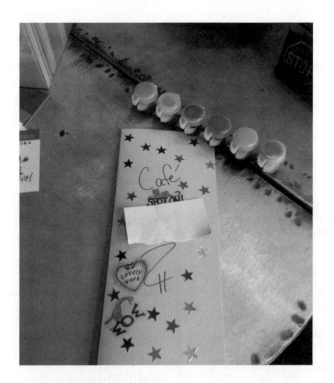

FIGURE 7.4. Front Cover of Sensory Menu.

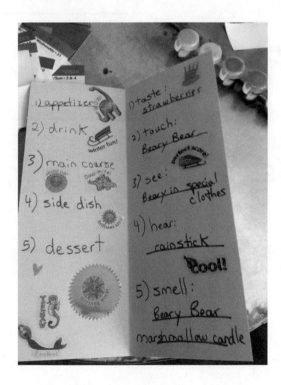

FIGURE 7.5. Example of Sensory Menu.

A SENSORY SOOTHING MENU

APPETIZER: Name a taste that helps you feel good and safe on the inside.

_____

BREAD BASKET: Name a smell that helps you feel good and safe on the inside.

_____

MAIN COURSE: Name something you like to touch, feel, or hold that helps you feel good and safe on the inside.

_____

SIDE DISH: Name a sound that helps you feel good and safe on the inside.

_____

DESSERT: Name a picture or visual image that helps you feel good and safe on the inside.

_____

FIGURE 7.6. Sensory Menu Template.

it exists alongside their child's limbic brain, the center of their emotional literacy. Children need training in naming and taming their emotions. This emotional literacy development begins in infancy and requires the support of the parent (Goleman, 2006; LeDoux, 1996). As a child emotes through cries, giggles, and shrieks, the good enough parent makes meaning of these communications. Take, for example, an infant who is sleeping peacefully when all of a sudden a large sanitation truck pulls up on the street outside the baby's bedroom window and a trash can makes an enormous crashing sound as it is picked up and dumped. The baby startles awake and begins to cry intensely, having trouble catching his breath between cries. The mother who is focused wholly on soothing the baby will run up the stairs, scoop him up, and begin to bounce and soothe him, saying, "Shhh, shhh, shhh, it's OK." The baby will calm down, and soon all will be at peace. The mother who is dually focused on both soothing the baby's physiology and enhancing emotional vocabulary will still run up the stairs, scoop up the baby, and begin to rock and soothe him, but may instead offer verbiage something like this: "It's OK. That big loud sound scared you. You were sleeping so peacefully, and all of a sudden there was a big, loud noise. That was so scary, but you're safe now. Mommy's got you." The baby will calm and all will be at peace, but the feedback loop will have now included learning aimed at the whole brain—soothing for the reptilian brain stem, matching of affect for the limbic brain, and words for feelings aimed at the neocortex—giving words to describe the full-body input that the baby is receiving from the lower brain regions (see Figure 7.7).

In Figure 7.7, the first response is aimed simply at quieting and reassuring the child, a typical goal for parents. This response may become the most urgent goal when the piercing cries of the child trigger the parent's own sympathetic nervous system and the parent's equilibrium is threatened. However, the second response

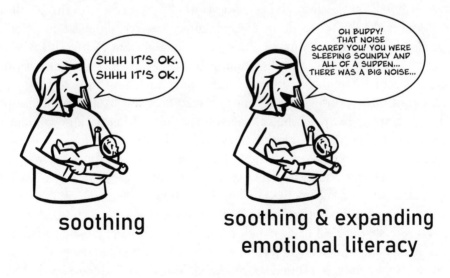

FIGURE 7.7. Soothing While Expanding Emotional Literacy.

will most likely accomplish the goal of quieting and reassuring the child (especially if delivered in modulated tones and with empathy), while also expanding the emotional literacy of the child by (1) giving words to the emotion that the child is experiencing and (2) tying the emotional response to a specific situation. We keep blank copies of this cartoon that have empty thought bubbles in large quantities at Nurture House. When a parent brings up a scenario in which naming the feelings involved in a child's escalation may have helped the parent and child remain more attuned, while helping the parent organize the child's experience in a way that honors bottom-up brain development, we can assist him or her in crafting another response. We find that offering concrete tools to a parent for a role-play redo of their response in a given situation sets the stage for application to situations that will come up in the future. It also serves as another support of the parallel process we encourage in family systems. The parent gets to participate in a redo by first crafting the response on paper and then practicing in a full-body role-play with the therapist, encouraging the mom or dad to recap what happened, connecting the event (e.g., a block tower collapsing) to an emotional state. Once two or three situations have been processed in session with the support of the therapist using this tool, additional blank copies of the cartoon can be sent home to support therapeutic homework. Clinicians can ask parents to identify just one moment within the week where they were able to verbally tie an emotional response to a situation that was emotionally challenging for the client, and fill in the cartoon with the language they used. The parent then brings this back to the next session for processing with the therapist.

As infants become toddlers, their mobility increases, they can cover more territory as they explore their environment, and parents continue to help their children make meaning of their expanding microcosm. Take, for example, the toddler who is building a tower with blocks on the kitchen floor several feet away from Mom. Mom is busily stirring a pot when she hears the crash. The toddler begins to shriek and pound her hands on the ground. Dad, who is wholly focused on soothing will run over and say, "It's OK. You're all right." Dad's affect may be calm, his tone soft and/or cheerful, hoping to cajole his daughter into a state of calm. While this response may be intended to de-escalate the child, it could also be incongruent with how the child is actually feeling, and if her emotional state is not validated by the parent as part of his response, soothing may ultimately be less likely. Dad might pick her up and comfort her until she calms and may then set her back down, redirect the toddler's attention to the blocks, stack one of the blocks on top of another to demonstrate, and hand a block to the toddler to do the same. Once the toddler is reengaged in play, the dad shifts his focus back to helping Mom prepare dinner.

The dad who is dually focused on soothing and expanding emotional literacy will offer a different kind of feedback. When the toddler shrieks, this dad will still rush over to help, but he'll likely match the child's affect more closely and attempt to mirror the child's intensity of feeling with his voice while he scoops the toddler up, saying, "Oh, buddy, you sound so frustrated! You worked so hard on that block tower and then, when you were just about to make it taller, it all fell down. I would be frustrated, too." The parent interprets the emotion that the child is feeling. The feeling may be frustration, it may be disappointment—the nuance of feeling words is expanded over time, but naming emotions, even if you are beginning with categories of emotion, and even if you don't name with 100% accuracy every time, is vastly superior to leaving the child in a vacuum of information. In this second scenario, dad is holding and soothing the toddler, but also naming her feeling and tying it to the hard work he observed and the devastation she feels at the demise of the block structure. Mirroring her distress communicates to the toddler that Dad sees her, feels her, . . . and ultimately (although 2-year-olds don't yet have this phraseology) gets her.

Clinicians can use the above examples as role-play scenarios in session as they are helping parents hone these emotional literacy skills for their children. After much trial and error with our families at Nurture House, we have realized that while we constantly hold the focus of supporting bottom-up brain development for both child and adult members of the system, parents are often soothed by approaching new patterns of response in a top-down way. Parents are thus frequently soothed by head knowledge. It feels natural and normal for them to engage in an exchange of ideas with another grown-up. This traditional talk format—sharing the ideas that we want to embed in the parent both verbally and with some form of a visual aid, some sort of recording tool—meets parents in their thinking brain and speaks to their executive function, respecting the parents' desire to reflect on concepts and their application to the daily experience of their child while building rapport. It is important all along the way that the clinician assign positive intentionality to the current response patterns being established by the parents with the child client, while working hard to genuinely enjoy the parents. The parallel process that TraumaPlay therapists hold as a core mechanism in our work begins as the clinician delights in the parents, giving a dose of what we will be asking them to give to their child.

Once the parent's thinking brain has been engaged and she has had supported time to plan and rehearse her response, the interactions concretized in the cartoons in Figure 7.7 can be role-played live between therapist and parent in session. Parents sometimes feel awkward about role-plays, but the full-body practice of them, pushing through the awkwardness (translated as potential arousal of the sympathetic nervous system), will allow for the healthy, titrated parasympathetic nervous system responses to be practiced with the supportive presence of the therapist. We want parents to practice enough that they will be able to remain grounded when they begin responding differently at home with their children. Clinicians should make the first couple of practices pretty easy for the parent so that they can experience a competency surge. The bar can then be raised slightly, with the understanding that parents may then feel adrift or begin to get overwhelmed in the midst of a role-play. They might begin to move into a frozen or sluggish response pattern. This is a good thing when it shows up, as it is likely to mirror their physiological responses when they are unsure how to respond to their child at home. Part of what the clinician is hoping to do is to bring, in small, incremental, manageable steps, the distress the parent feels when dealing with the child into the active moments of engagement with the therapist: In other words, we are hoping to bring the parent's problematic neurophysiological responses—those that they experience with the identified child client—into the room with the therapist first so that we can begin to address them.

In another parallel process, parents need to experience us as safely in charge of the clinical space in order to risk trying out new behaviors, applying new thoughts, and experiencing new emotional connections with their children. We are asking parents to expand their Safe Boss skills set with their own children, and the first step in this process is that we remain regulated and grounded during our interactions with parents. When a parent shows up with overwhelming feelings of helplessness or hopelessness, it is possible for the clinician to experience a sense of helplessness themself. Therapists must cultivate a duality of self in order to be with parents in their distress while not entering into the hopeless emotion or narrative themselves. This duality is ultimately what we are asking parents to cultivate, and we must lead the way. If parents are to be helpful to the child in the vortex, it is important that we don't get swept up into it with them. The concept is a confusing one: We are asking parents to simultaneously validate their child's big feelings without entering into them.

The therapeutic community can take for granted the skills of unconditional positive regard, assigning positive intentionality and validating the experience of your client before offering anything else, but most caregivers (parents, teachers, day care workers) have not had the luxury of direct instruction and coached practice of these skills sets. Most parents need support in learning that holding a child's big feeling and reflecting it can be defusing.

The observation of a play session can generate a wealth of information with regard to the feeling states that can be tolerated by the parent and those that cannot. Sometimes parents have trouble tolerating a feeling that their child is displaying because they have previous negative associations with the display of this emotion. Picture Jessica, a 33-year-old mother of three. When Jessica was a little girl, her mother was depressed and her father worked all the time. Starting in the second grade, Jessica went to school on her own, came home alone, did her homework, and made dinner for the family. Sometimes her mom couldn't get off the couch, and Jessica would caretake her; bringing her water, telling her jokes, and rubbing her feet. Every now and then, Jessica could get her mother to laugh, but other times nothing she did seemed to help. Her helplessness stemmed from being quietly assigned adult tasks and being quietly asked to take care of the adults when she couldn't possibly have the tools she needed to do that job well as a child. She was supposed to be taken care of, not assume the role of the caretaker. Jessica learned how to squash her own feelings, perform well, and monitor other people's feelings. Fast forward, with Jessica feeling overwhelmed and resentful when her little girl seems sad or has big needs. It triggers that little girl part of Jessica that felt unequipped (and rightly so) to caretake as a child. This mother is likely to require some therapeutic support that guides her toward an expansion of self-compassion so that she has more compassion to give to her daughter. How do we do that? Slowly, as we help Jessica grow reflective capacity around her own attachment relationship with her mother. The younger parts of her self resonate with the sadness and associate it with her mother's depression. Jessica's mission when she was a child was to pull her mom out of sadness so that Jessica could get her own needs met by an unavailable mom. Jessica still believes that sadness is dangerous, both because it may take her daughter away from her and because she feels helpless, perhaps even frozen, in the face of it. Jessica may try to cajole her daughter into being happy, much like she would try to cajole her mother out of sadness.

Several years ago, I worked with Timothy, a 10-year-old boy who had survived brain cancer. He had been through multiple rounds of chemo and radiation and was now in remission. His parents were committed to his care, and his mother was always the one to take him to doctors' appointments and to remain with him overnight when he had to stay in the hospital. His hair had begun to grow back like peach fuzz, and his mother was often stroking his head when I went out to greet him in the lobby. In their dyadic session, Timothy and his mom appeared connected. When she told a story about him as a baby, her eyes welled up with tears, and he reached out to touch her hand and said, "It's OK, Mom." It wasn't until we had completed several individual sessions that Timothy was able to begin giving me a glimpse into his inner life. I had wondered if he carried some underlying anxiety related to all the medical procedures. I drew a gingerbread outline of a person (as I often do, since my drawing skills are remedial at best) and then offered Timothy the Anxiety Buttons activity (a variation of the Anger Buttons exercise [Goodyear-Brown, 2002]). He pushed the buttons away and asked for markers. I moved the markers in front of him. He thought about what he would draw for a minute and then he chose an orange marker and drew a heart with eyes, a nose, and a mouth in the shape of a frown. He then drew a type of arrow pointing to the image (in case I had perhaps missed it?). I said, "Tell me about that," gesturing to the heart. He replied, "That's my heart. His name is Hidey Hearty." I repeated the name, and we both looked at the drawing for a moment. Then Timothy said, "Yeah, it's the heart that hides." I was blown away. This little person had gotten very skilled at hiding his big feelings. Although I did not yet understand all the dynamics of the parent–child system, I wondered if he had sensed his mother's distress when he expressed pain or fear or sadness, so he had learned to modulate his expression while he was going through all those medical procedures. Timothy took his art home with him that day, but I have since had occasion to re-create Hidey Hearty for other clients. He has become an invaluable tool for beginning to help parents understand how children might modulate their emotional expression in order to remain connected to the caregiver without overwhelming him or her, a primal attachment behavior that enables the child to stay close to the parent, especially in times of great upheaval or threat (see Figure 7.8).

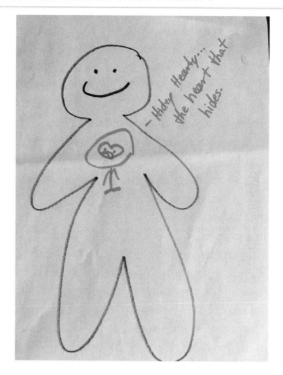

FIGURE 7.8. The Hidey Hearty.

The Color-Your-Heart activity (Goodyear-Brown, 2002) has become a go-to assessment tool in TraumaPlay, in part because it quantifies a large amount of emotional information quickly, and in part because it helps to shape a parent's perceptions of their child's inner emotional life very early on in treatment. Parents often need a paradigm shift from "my child is angry all the time" to an awareness that anger is the most powerful feeling—and therefore the easiest to share when the child is under stress—but may actually be another "Hidey Hearty" phenomenon: Only this time, the child's true heart is hidden under a continual veneer of anger or irritation. Sometimes parents begin to make this shift after they see that half of the child's Color-Your-Heart is consumed with worry, or fear, or loneliness. As parents compare this quantification to their child's behaviors, they begin to see that the underlying emotional motivation is usually more vulnerable.

Duality of Anger

A similar shift occurs when parents and children who share an emotional display or propensity that leans toward anger begin to explore the other, more vulnerable feelings that often engender anger. In Figure 7.9, you will find two Anger Volcanoes: one created by a teenage son, the other by his parent. The family was referred because some of its members weren't as connected as the parents wanted them to be, and

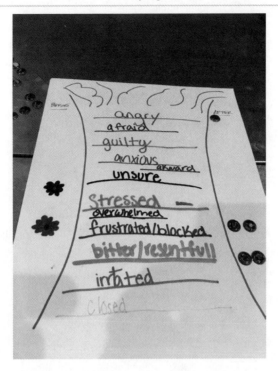

FIGURE 7.9. Teenager's Anger Volcano.

the primary emotional expression of several family members was irritation or frustration. I used Mixed-Emotion Cards to help the teen begin identifying the feelings underneath his anger. Notice in Figure 7.9 that these underlying feelings included being guilty, unsure, stressed, anxious, overwhelmed, and bitter. I was also curious about the parent's experience of anger and asked the parent to create a personal Anger Volcano, too. I again offered the Mixed-Emotion Cards and again found that emotions such as being overwhelmed, disappointed, worried, and stressed showed up as more vulnerable feelings underlying the anger (see Figure 7.10). I asked both the parent and the teen to enter into a week's work of becoming more aware of their feelings either prior to a behavioral eruption in frustration or even in the wake of it. I offered both family members a set of stickers and asked them to just put stickers next to the feelings they could identify, either before or after a moment of expressed anger. In the teenager's case, the general feeling of stress was associated with anger expression, and for the parent a sense of disappointment was associated with anger. This first week's worth of information established a shared understanding within the family that more vulnerable feelings can be communicated, and help can be offered by other family members, before toxic anger expression takes over.

Parents and children can also work together on understanding that it's possible to have several different emotions all at the same time. The Mixed-Emotion Cards can be a useful tool for helping them comprehend this as well. I will sit with parents and children and lay out the Mixed-Emotion Cards just like I would if I was playing

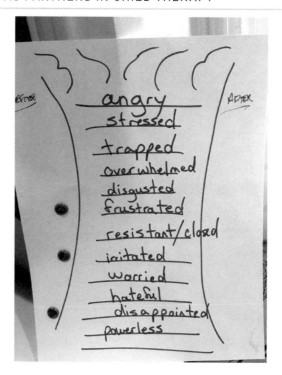

FIGURE 7.10. Parent's Anger Volcano.

a game of Memory. We then discuss a family memory (always beginning with easier memories and only eventually moving to harder content). I offer a large basket of colored stones and invite the child first and then the parent to choose handfuls of stones to place on any emotion that they had in relation to the memory we identified. Sometimes parents and children have shared emotional experiences, and certain cards end up with stones from both parent and child covering the image. In other cases, either the parent or the child gets to learn that the other experienced a different set of emotions or a different intensity of the same emotions in relation to the same event (see Figure 7.11).

When It Gets Complicated

With some of our most complex little ones, the sensory experiences are encoded on an emotional level and emotions can be encoded on a sensory level. The drawing offered in Figure 7.12 is the best example of this complex presentation I have been able to find. An elementary-school-age child who has dealt with a combination of sensory defensive and sensory seeking intensities his whole life, while also asking the core questions ("Am I good?" "Am I loved?" "Do I have a place in the world?"), caught a cold. He didn't feel well physically. His mom kept him home from school, and he spent the time making the drawing you see in Figure 7.12. He is a very bright

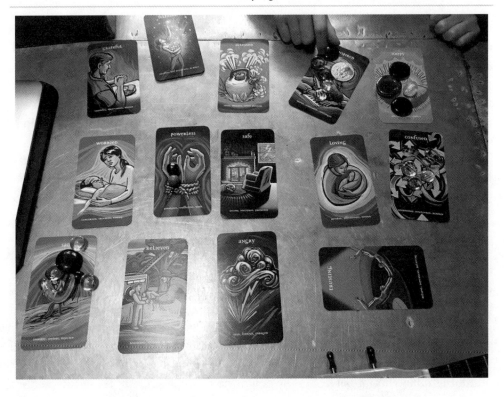

FIGURE 7.11. Two Emotional Reactions to the Same Event.

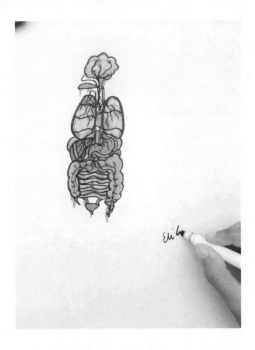

FIGURE 7.12. Insides Melting.

boy and has frequently drawn internal anatomy for me, but on this day he drew his own physiology, but with all the organs, beginning with his brain and moving all the way down into his pelvis, bleeding. He asked his mother if he could send this picture to me, and when she asked him what he wanted to call it, he said, "I feel like my insides are melting." I don't believe that this was experienced on a purely sensory or a purely emotional level, but presented an astonishing interweaving of somatic experiences and feelings.

Once parents understand more about how to support their child's reptilian regulation needs, his limbic emotional literacy needs, and needs for connection, the therapist can spend some time helping the parents become more aware of the same child's thought life, the way that thought life interfaces with their emotions and actions, and how their own cognitions and those of their child might interface. We just touch on this work here by referencing the cognitive triangle that we introduce to both parents and children. Thoughts, feelings, and behaviors are intimately connected for each of us (Goodyear-Brown, 2010a). Where it gets especially complicated is when the thoughts of a parent engender certain feelings and behaviors in relation to their child . . . and then the child's thoughts about the parent's behavior show up in their own feelings and actions in relation to that parent. This overlap of a child's cognitive triad with a parent's cognitive triad is happening continuously, and for families that are able to slow down the process, some of these interactions can be teased out. To this end, templates of a child's cognitive triangle (see Figure 7.13) and a slightly larger parent's cognitive triangle (see Figure 7.14) are included here. Brave clinicians can identify a parenting moment that went off the rails and explore the thoughts, feelings, and actions of parent and child. In some cases, a powerful representation of the interconnection of these familial processes becomes clear when you overlay the child's triangle upside down on top of the parent's triangle. What we end up with is a star that holds the thoughts, feelings, and behaviors of both parent and child in relation to a difficult family event. Our cognitions are the formation of story and define selfhood.

The Child's Cognitive Triangle

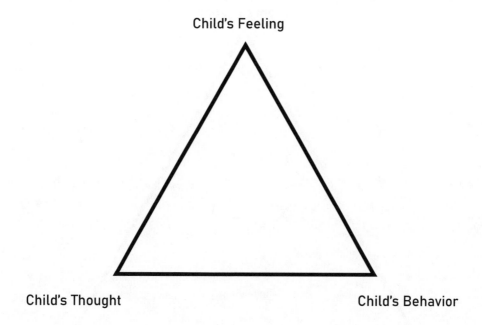

Child's Feeling

Child's Thought

Child's Behavior

Describe a time when you acted in a way that you weren't proud of.

FIGURE 7.13. Child's Cognitive Triangle.

The Parent's Cognitive Triangle

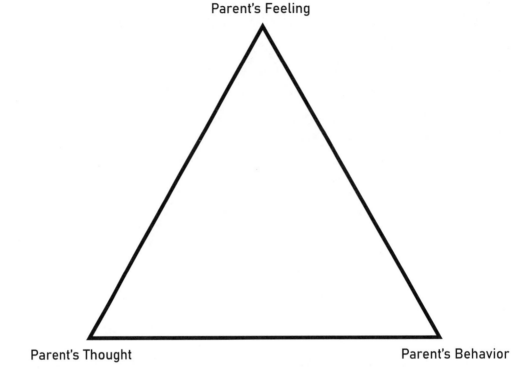

Parent's Feeling

Parent's Thought

Parent's Behavior

Describe a time when you acted in a way that you weren't proud of.

FIGURE 7.14. Parent's Cognitive Triangle.

CHAPTER 8

Helping Parents Set Boundaries and Deal with Big Behaviors

Quick on the heels of validating big emotions comes the need to provide healthy boundaries around how these emotions are managed and expressed. Children feel safest when they know both the limits and that their safe bosses can enforce the limits. When parents are easily overwhelmed, the children end up feeling more powerful than their parents. When children end up feeling they have more power than their parents, they begin to feel very unsafe—particularly when they are experiencing their own loss of control and no one is able to mitigate this or hem them in.

Messy Work

The majority of therapists would agree that marital therapy is not interchangeable with parent coaching or co-parent work, but these same therapists would also agree that the lines get really blurry and messy at times. Child therapists often end up dealing with core relational issues in the marriage by virtue of the deeply held feelings, beliefs, and communications between two adult partners about parenting practices. Whatever problematic communication patterns exist are often exacerbated by the stresses of parenting. Most moms and dads genuinely want the best for their children, and when what they believe to be best for their child isn't upheld or embraced by their partner, co-parents end up communicating their needs in dysfunctional ways.

Child therapists are often wary of stepping on land mines of anger, resentment, abandonment, judgment, vying needs for power and control when they work with parents, especially parents who are not currently parenting on the same page.

The action steps and psychoeducation involved in helping parents work through trigger points may change based on the point of disagreement, but this impasse is often a snapshot of the larger ways in which each parent approaches their adult partner as well as their children. It can be difficult when a clinician is first entering a parenting system to discern where the differences lie. Each parent may have different kinds of hooks, and it will be helpful to both parents if these hooks become known within the system. If there are two parents, more than likely there are differences in their permissiveness, and this will also require honest exploration. Let's start with hooks.

The Hook

So much is happening under the surface of what we perceive in the communication exchange between parents and children. There are loops of communication that happen between parent and child over and over again. This can be both good and not-so-good news for dyads. Children naturally engage in attachment-grounded proximity-seeking behaviors. Parents and children can have lots of loving moments together when the parent is grounded and present, but the parent is unable to offer these same loving responses when they are activated. There are several exercises that can help parents begin to explore more fully how they become triggered by their children. Many parent–therapist conversations are focused on the child's worst behaviors. Questions such as "Which of your child's behaviors is most triggering for you?" are often heard during the assessment phase of treatment. What if we turn this on its head and begin to instead look at self with the parent? What if our question became "When you have had your worst parenting moments . . . the ones where you don't like how you are behaving and you wish you could take it back, what was happening between you and your child?" The way we ask questions, the way we wonder about various parts of the family system, begins to lay the groundwork for more mentalization and deeper reflection. Our children are more likely to trigger the unhealed parts of self than any other relationship in our adult lives.

The parts of self that experience pain when feeling out of control are mightily triggered by our children, who will push back against control in order to individuate. Children enter this world a gorgeous mess of innocence, vulnerability, and disorganization. Any parent who has ever swaddled the infant who is flailing about with a beet red face while crying uncontrollably, unable to make the transition from wake to sleep but desperately in need of sleep, can attest to the organizing function the parent provides. When babies are hungry, they cry to be fed; when they need a hug, they cry to be picked up. These displays of distress are perfectly healthy proximity-seeking attachment behaviors. But for the mom who has her own unresolved hurt, who experienced food insecurity as a child, or who had no one to hold her when she needed it, the earliest attachment wounds in the parent become triggered by the child's displays of attachment behavior. In a healthy parent–child dyad, the child expresses need and the parent meets it. If the child expresses a need over and over again and the parent seems disinterested, angry, or overwhelmed by the need, the child begins developing his defenses. After repeated attempts by the toddler to elicit care, through coming closer and lifting his arms, asking to be held by a mom who struggles with postpartum depression, the toddler will begin to prioritize the mother's needs above his own.

Early childhood is a time of natural egocentricity. Babies are born with an unwavering mission to stay alive, and they can't yet do anything for themselves, so the focus must be on inviting, enticing, or training the grown-ups around them to provide all that they need. Their tools are limited but powerful. Babies are born soft-wired with attachment capacities and a whole vocabulary for how to get their needs met. Cries, giggles, coos, toothless grins, raging shrieks—each of these is part of the baby's vocabulary for need meeting. However, which parts of this early attachment vocabulary become hard-wired, which are abandoned, and which are replaced with miscues have to do with how these proximity-seeking displays are received by the caregiver. When we first enter this world, regulation occurs almost exclusively within relationship. The most formative experiences in which a baby perceives relationship as regulating are moments when relationship is paired with resource. For example, when the baby is hungry, she cries for her mother who comes and picks her up to feed. The breast or the bottle provides the actual nutrients that fuel the baby, but these nutrients are paired with the snuggled embrace, loving strokes, lilting, high-frequency motherese, and the loving eye gaze of the parent. The baby feels satisfied, satiated afterward because her emotional and somatic needs for connection have been met, while the resource of food has been dispensed. Moving from this understanding that regulation is found in our earliest relationships, we often talk with parents about being the neurobiological co-regulators of their children. However, these are just fancy words and don't take into account that, while the parent is meant to lead, the parent and child are mutually co-regulating . . . or dysregulating each other.

Using the handout labeled "Which of Your Child's Behaviors Hook You?" (Figure 8.1), ask each parent to list the top three behaviors that, when the child engages in them, quickly hook the parent into an escalated response. These might include eye rolling, deep sighing, ignoring directions, slamming doors, and so on. This activity can be particularly fun to do with both parents in the same session. The therapist invites them to fill out the handout separately and then they compare notes.

How Are You Viewing Behavior?

Once the hooks have been identified, we want to get at the cognitive distortion that is being triggered in the parent. In addition to actual sunglasses on which a parent can write, we offer the handout in Figure 8.2. Two pairs of glasses are offered. The

WHICH OF YOUR CHILD'S BEHAVIORS HOOK YOU?

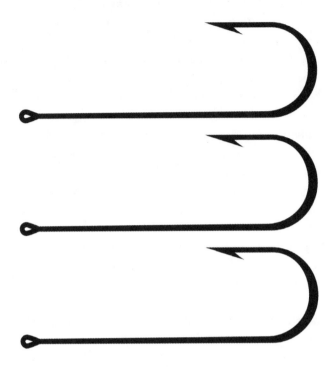

WRITE THE TOP THREE HOOK-WORTHY BEHAVIORS ON THE HOOKS PROVIDED ABOVE

FIGURE 8.1. What Hooks You?

first pair represents the parent's first thought about the behavior, their interpretation at first glance. The second pair represents a potential reframe of the behavior in terms of an underlying need of the child: These lenses require pulling back to a larger view and seeing the bigger picture. This might involve helping parents look at antecedents to the moment of the big behavior. It might require them to check in with themselves about the basic regulation needs of the child. Has he eaten? Been given proper hydration? Slept? Had sensory needs met?

What would happen if instead of seeing the explanation "He's doing it for attention!" as a negative, somehow dark motivation, we understood it with relief,

HOW ARE YOU VIEWING BEHAVIOR?

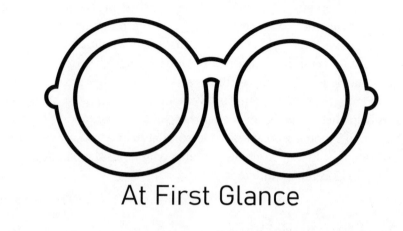

At First Glance

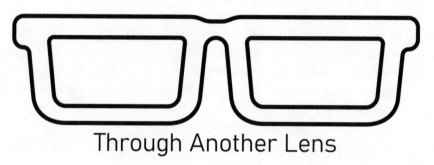

Through Another Lens

FIGURE 8.2. How Are You Viewing Behavior?

thinking to ourselves, "Well, if more intentional doses of attention or connection are what he needs, we can give that to him!" Replacing the negative thought bubble "He is doing that for attention" with "He is really needing connection" shifts us away from perceiving manipulation in his behavior to perceiving his behavior as expressing a need. Then our job as the Safe Boss is to help him ask for what he needs with his authentic voice. One of the first things I do with parents who are here assigning negative motives to their children is use this handout (see Figure 8.2). Once we have identified the child's hooking behaviors, we can examine them one by one and help parents reflect on their own process for interpreting these behaviors. Using the glasses at the top of the handout, the parent writes in her first, knee-jerk response to a behavior. The child delays obedience and the parent immediately thinks, "He is trying to make me upset!" The parent writes this first-glance interpretation in the first pair of glasses. The act of writing it down begins to bring a little perspective to the thought, and then the parent and clinician can explore other alternatives together. Perhaps the child needs more help focusing his attention. Perhaps there were several people in the room, and the child would benefit from the parent saying his name and making eye contact before giving the direction. Usually, several explanations of behavior might be investigated once a parent has acknowledged her initial interpretation. We might provide any of the psychoeducation, Reflective Attachment Work, or Storykeeping for the Parent that is needed to help the parent begin seeing the child through another lens. As we work together we fashion a second set of glasses that help encode whatever somatic strategies, paradigm shifts, or co-regulation understandings the parent needs to see and meet the child's behavior differently.

Laying Down New Neural Wiring

Much of the way that parents view behavior is focused on what they want their children to stop doing. They want their children to stop yelling, lying, or being self-ish. I usually begin, even in the intake session, helping parents begin to shift their paradigm from a view toward what they want to squelch to a view of what they want to grow. I will explain that the brain is like tall grass: If you walk across it once, it

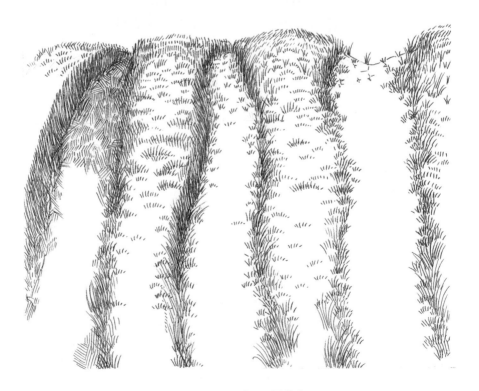

FIGURE 8.3. Paths in Tall Grass.

bounces right back; if you walk across it again and again, you lay down new pathways (Hebb, 1949). This metaphor for neuroplasticity (Jackson, 1958; Kay, 2009; Mundkur, 2005; Siegel, 2010) often helps parents (or teachers) refocus on what they want to see more of. I offer the beautiful drawing shown in Figure 8.3 and begin to ask parents what sorts of behaviors they want to see laid down in their children's neural wiring.

We then offer the "Neural Pathways" handout (see Figure 8.4) and help parents go deeper in terms of defining an adaptive neural pathway that is already deeply ingrained. An example: He can already ask for what he needs when he needs it. We then ask the parent to identify a neural pathway that the child has started to lay down, but that requires support from the parent. An example: He will brush his teeth each morning and night with a reminder from me. Finally, we ask the parent

Neural Pathways

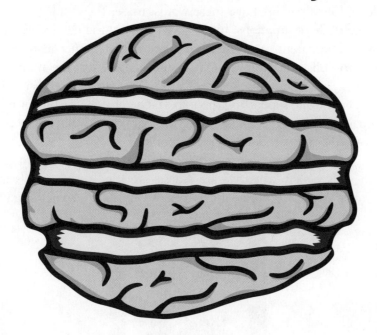

Write in the most worn path a behavior that your child has already mastered. Then identify one that they are still working on, and one that you will need to intentionally practice to lay down new or deeper neural pathways.

FIGURE 8.4. Neural Pathways.

to identify a neural pathway (tied to a behavior) that she wants to see her child lay down, but that she sees very little daily evidence of at this point in the child's development. An example: I want him to ask permission before turning on the TV. Each of these behaviors are written into the three pathways on the handout of pathways in the brain.

House Rules and a Culture of Kindness

Stick together. Have fun. No hurts. Simple rules under which many other rules can be housed. I first heard these rules at a Theraplay training; we applied these three basic rules at Camp Nurture, and they are also the posted rules of Nurture House (see Figure 8.5).

To my mind, the most important of these rules is stick together. It is together that fears are calmed. It is together that nonverbal cues can be read. It is together that problems are solved. It is together that we feel seen, heard, and know that we are not alone. Once parents have these words inside, they find themselves using them in a multitude of situations. In the grocery store, the child starts to run into another aisle. The parent says, "Remember, we stick together in here!" When a child begins to pull away from a mom in the parking lot, the normal response is "Stop!," "No!," or "Come back here." Stick together offers a positively worded reminder instead, while supporting the importance of the attachment relationship as a continual safety anchor. Family is the first team that children experience. The phrase *stick together* reinforces this team mentality.

Even when we disagree, we stick together. Even when we are in distress, we stick together. Especially when we are scared, we stick together. When there is something to be celebrated, we do it together. When there is something hard to do,

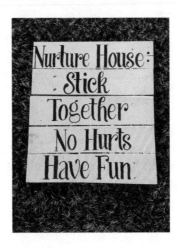

FIGURE 8.5. Nurture House Rules.

we do it together. The harder it is, the more we stick like glue. We have multiple activities at Nurture House that help children and their parents learn and practice these rules until they become part of the family's lexicon and, more importantly, part of the family's culture. Emotional hurts, verbal hurts, and physical hurts all fall under the "No hurts" rule, and the mitigator of all discipline is having fun together because the more relationally full the parent and child feel with one another, the more discipline will feel like a blip on the radar screen. Sometimes parents have trouble making a quick correction and then returning to fun, feeling almost like the withholding of affection or connection through play should be the consequence and will create a good learning opportunity. Helping parents understand that shared fun is actually preemptive discipline may take some time. We have families develop their own set of rules together. Often families choose to use the Nurture House rules, but there is extra room on the worksheet for families to add an additional rule if there is a specific growing edge that we want to see the family grow into. This worksheet can be found later in the chapter in Figure 8.9.

Ice Cubes

My friend and colleague Amy Frew created this intervention. Here is the idea: The clinician takes several ice cubes fresh out of the freezer (at least a couple need to be really cold) and asks the parent and child to make them stick together. Very cold ice cubes can be stacked on top of each other but will slip off of each other immediately. Wait a couple of minutes and try again. As the ice cubes begin to melt the tiniest bit, they stick together—there's a powerful metaphor in that. As both parent and child become less rigid (but who are we kidding, it will have to be the parent first), it is easier for the parent and child to be a team and stick together.

The Static Stick

This tried-and-true experiment helps reinforce the "stick together" rule . . . with a twist. We all know that when you take a balloon and rub it against someone's head vigorously, static electricity is created. This is fun and funny in its own right, and often leads to the parent, child, and therapist all sharing a moment of delight and silliness (which we know releases oxytocin, the bonding chemical) and enhances our bonds with one another. Once the static electricity has been created, the balloon will usually stick to our hair, our clothes, and sometimes the walls! This is perceived as almost magical by children, but for the grown-ups who know how static electricity is created, we understand that friction is the main ingredient. This is a powerful metaphor, too, since the moments at which a parent is giving the reminder to stick together are usually times of friction between parent and child.

Stick Together Bookmarks

We keep many varieties of duct tape stored in a clear jar at Nurture House. The therapist invites the parent and child to explore all of them and to each choose a pattern or color. Parent and child measure the same amount of tape from each of their choices and stick the two pieces together to form bookmarks. As we make them, we talk about a unique characteristic of the child and of the parent (see Figure 8.6 and Figure 8.7).

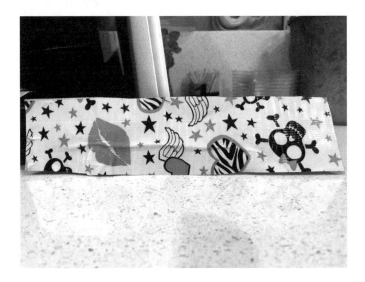

FIGURE 8.6. Child's Chosen Pattern.

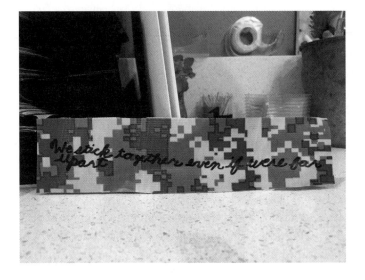

FIGURE 8.7. Parent's Chosen Pattern.

Stick Together Game

A set of building toys called Squigz revolutionized my practice for a period of time. Especially for children, the perfect prop can help them grasp a concept that might otherwise be difficult to comprehend. The manufacturer Fat Brain Toys refers to the toys as "Fun Little Suckers!" They are fun. Each piece has a bendable middle with one suction cup at each end. Some are short, and some are long. The larger pieces can be pressed between the forehead of a parent and child and bring their noses within a couple of inches of each other. Longer connections can be made to give parent and child more room to maneuver but still keeps them stuck together! Figure 8.8 is a photograph of my sister-in-law Whitney and me sticking together on the streets of Charleston, South Carolina. In the playroom, I offer the pieces to a parent and child, and once they are stuck together, I ask them to move to another part of the room or to accomplish a playful task without breaking the physical connection they have established. With older children and teens, I process what was difficult about the activity afterward. This can lead to some surprisingly rich conversation uncovering some of the core difficulties such a system poses in maintaining connection and individual autonomy while moving through life together (see Figure 8.8).

Magnets

Using a large stack of shiny metallic magnetic rocks, have parent and child explore the attraction and repulsion properties of the rocks together. If you turn two rocks in the same direction, their polarity pushes them apart. Children will try to push the two stones together and will feel the tension, an invisible force field, that continually results in the two stones moving away from each other. We then turn them so that their polarities attract each other. This force can be so strong it becomes difficult to pull apart the two stones. At Nurture House, we have a metallic table in our sand tray room. Parents and children enjoy putting one of the magnetic rocks on the underside of the table and one on top of the table. When you move the rock underneath, it makes the rock on top move, as if by magic. We talk about how, when we stick together, we can do magical and powerful things. This can also be a metaphor for the invisible force that continues to exist between parent and child when they are apart.

It is my deep belief that families who play together, stay together. In our family, we turn on blasting music and dance around the kitchen while we are putting away groceries, not every time but enough times that we have all developed a sense that doing the hard thing is easier when we are doing it together. As family rules are being developed, it is well worth asking which of the family chores are most worth doing together; If playfulness can be intertwined in the task, it gets done more

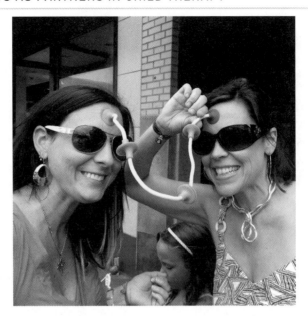

FIGURE 8.8. Stick Together Squigz Connector.

quickly while reinforcing the message that together we can do hard things. The "Family Rules Worksheet" (see Figure 8.9) can serve as an anchor as families are exploring the culture they want to create in their home.

Parents often work very hard to make things fair in families. Finding the parent's key cognitive distortions in relation to their parenting is also critically important. One of the core distortions that a parent may carry is that good parents make sure everything is fair. If Manuel gets 20 minutes of screen time, so does Maria. If Manuel gets to stay up until 9 P.M., so should Maria. We replace the statement "In our family, everything is fair" with "In our family, everyone gets what they need." Sometimes a short, simple mantra that the family can absorb is the fastest way to combatting and eventually shifting key cognitive distortions. One of our guideposts at Nurture House is this statement: "In our family, everyone gets *all* of what we need and *some* of what we want" (the mantra you see in Figure 8.10, one that we print out for clients).

As clinicians engage parents around what it means to meet each family member's needs and say "yes" to some of what they want, our conversations go deeper. Manuel has a term paper due on Friday, and he needs to work on it for 2 hours a night after his baseball practice ends. He will be staying up until 10 P.M. Maria is 4 years younger, needs more sleep, and has a school day that starts earlier than her brother's. Her bedtime is 8 P.M., with 30 minutes of snuggle time and book reading built in with Mom. Both children get all of what they need. Additionally, Mom may realize that the term paper work requires a lot of focus and decide to give Manuel 20 minutes of screen time after his schoolwork, even though it's kind of late, because the activity will be comforting. In the same way, Mom may decide to read one more

Family Rules Worksheet

What do we want more of in our family?

What do we want less of in our family?

What rules do we need to help us get there?

1)

2)

3)

Family Rules:

1) In our family, we do

2) In our family, we don't

3)

4)

FIGURE 8.9. Family Rules Worksheet.

> ## IN OUR FAMILY,
> ### EVERYONE GETS **ALL** OF
> ### WHAT WE *need*
> ### AND **SOME** OF WHAT WE
> # *want.*

FIGURE 8.10. Family Mantra.

picture book to Maria as a way to give her an extra 10 minutes of connection since her bedtime is so much earlier.

Family sessions are often useful in working out the practical application of this mantra. We have a "Needs versus Wants Worksheet" (see Figure 8.11) that we use when we are beginning to introduce this idea to families. We give a copy to each family member. We talk about how everyone needs water in order to live, and how we like to drink all sorts of other things as well. Each child/teen can decide what kind of drink goes into the other cup with the straw. Sometimes it becomes a strawberry milkshake, other times a Coca-Cola. Most kids are willing to acknowledge that if they had milkshakes or Coca-Cola non-stop, they would feel pretty yucky, dehydrated, and have unnaturally high blood sugar. Therefore, the balance is that you get all of what you need (more water on days where you need extra fluids) and some of what you want. Each family member is given time to draw symbols inside the water bottle for the things they identify as needs in their family and time to draw symbols inside the paper cup to represent the additional wants that family members can sometimes say "yes" to.

At Nurture House, we find sand tray work to be very helpful in teasing out the difference between needs and wants. Family members are each given a small round sand tray and invited to fill it with miniatures that represent their individual wants and needs. We then offer them one larger sand tray to create together. Most families find that if they dump all of their wants and needs icons into the sand tray, it looks and feels like a chaotic mess. The exercise requires that all family members agree as to where each need is placed in the sand. Perhaps they agree that because they all chose icons for food, they can place all the food symbols in one area of the sand tray, or even use just one food symbol to represent this shared need of all family members. Each family member's symbols of wants also have to be negotiated and their placement within the tray agreed on by everyone. Rich conversations and some therapist-facilitated practice of negotiating how to meet needs can happen in this way.

NEEDS VS. WANTS

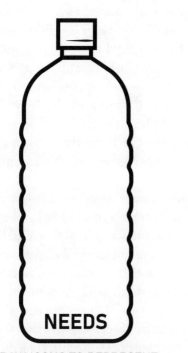
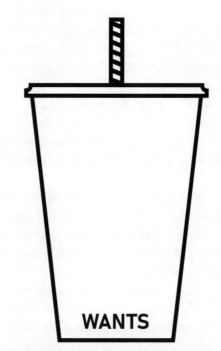

NEEDS

DRAW ICONS TO REPRESENT
THE BASIC NEEDS THAT FAMILY
CAN HELP YOU MEET.

WANTS

DRAW SYMBOLS TO REPRESENT
THE FUN STUFF, THE EXTRAS THAT YOU
SOMETIMES GET AS A MEMBER OF YOUR FAMILY.

FIGURE 8.11. Needs versus Wants.

Validate Feelings While Setting Limits

Parents often need to be shown how to validate feelings while still setting a limit. Sometimes parents believe that if they validate a child's feeling, it will take over all the space in the room and make setting a limit impossible. In fact, validating the big feeling helps to defuse it. Dan Siegel (2020) refers to this process as Name It to Tame It. If we point the parents back to their growing understanding of the triune brain, we can talk about this in terms of taking the limbic brain expression of emotion, articulating it linguistically, and therefore building a bridge from the lower limbic brain region to the neocortex, or thinking brain. Just this process can help leach the intensity out of an emotion. One of my favorite examples of attuning to and reflecting a child's deep emotion is given in the first edition of *How to Talk So Kids Will Listen and Listen So Kids Will Talk* by Adele Faber and Elaine Mazlish (1980/2012). They give a cartoon example of a child coming down for breakfast and wanting Cheerios. Unfortunately, the box of Cheerios is empty. The authors show two separate parenting responses. In the first, the parent acknowledges they are out of Cheerios and encourages the child to choose something else. The child escalates and the parent sets a limit on the behavior, but the child escalates to a full-scale tantrum. In the second response, the child demands Cheerios, and the parent matches what feels to the child like a desperate need for Cheerios, saying something like "I wish we had Cheerios for you . . . I wish we could fill up your whole crib with Cheerios" before setting a limit. Arguably, the wish fulfillment part of this response helps regulate the child, but more importantly, the parent gives weight to the feeling of loss and disappointment that the child is experiencing because there are no Cheerios.

Especially for children who come from hard places, want versus need balances on the head of a pin. When a child has grown up in an environment of lack, when a hard "no" is the response to a want, we can unintentionally kick that child's perception of a want into a need. The child with the core question "Will there be enough for me?" has difficulty with the hard "no." A soft "no" avoids the actual words *no, don't stop, quit,* and *not* (Hembree-Kigin & McNeil, 2013) and attempts to give some version of "yes" to the child. Some of that "yes" is given through the validation of feelings, validating that to the child it may feel necessary, whether the "it" is a granola bar or a toy that he just saw while checking out of the grocery store. Validating the intensity of the desire while still setting necessary limits can help the child remain connected to you.

Parenting Styles

The number and kinds of limits that get set in a family have to do with the parenting style of each parent. It is not unusual for parents to have very different parenting styles, and the executive subsystem may end up with defined roles of good cop/bad cop, which usually results in both parents feeling resentful after they have operated in their role for a period of time. Diana Baumrind's research (1989) on parenting styles influenced 40 years of parenting practice and created a typology for parenting in which parenting style fell into one of three categories: permissive, authoritarian, and authoritative. The permissive parent does not set boundaries with the child, allowing the child to be in charge of the house. The authoritarian parent is almost militaristic, communicates "It's my way or the highway," and leaves no room for negotiation or compromise. The authoritative parent, by contrast, is what we call the "Safe Boss" when we are training parents in discipline strategies for their children. These parents have some basic rules and boundaries but provide lots of room in the process for the child to speak. The parents will make the final decisions, but are happy to hear from their children with regard to their perceived wants, needs, and preferences. The children of authoritarian parents often become either overly submissive or rebellious. Children of permissive parents can become mini-narcissists, believing that their parents exist to serve them. These children do not internalize boundaries and have little respect for others. A balance of struc-ture and nurture in parenting produces children who know they are loved but are also respectful of the needs of others. A fourth category, uninvolved or neglectful parenting, is when a parent provides for basic needs but allows almost complete freedom, even when the allowed freedoms may place the child squarely in harm's way. These parents are often cold and unresponsive. They have no rules but also no nurture and they don't seem to care much what happens to their child. Children of these parents often end up with addictions or suicidal ideation or completion. The parenting styles grid (see Figure 8.12) helps parents think through where they fall on this continuum of structure and nurture. Offering copies of this grid to both parents can begin a reflective conversation about which quadrant each parent tends to operate in, how this affects their parenting subsystem, and whether or not there are tendencies either parent wants to work on changing.

Parents may also swing between extremes based on the amount of stress they are under; how much their parenting partner may be under- or overfunctioning; and other factors, such as whether or not in-laws with a different view of parenting are visiting. Another tool that we have introduced to parents is our "Parenting Pen-dulum" handout (see Figure 8.13), and it is the most fun to use as a take-home tool after playing with an actual pendulum, specifically a Newton's Cradle, in session. We have created stickers for each of the hanging weights—two each (one for each side) for the following descriptors: uninvolved, permissive, authoritative, aggressive, authoritarian. We like using the cradle because the movement and interaction of each ball with the others create force and influence. Each parent's parenting style affects the other's and the totality of the home environment.

Let's be honest. No one wants to be seen as authoritarian; it has become syn-onymous with dictatorial. In the same way, very few people want to be considered

WHERE ARE YOU?

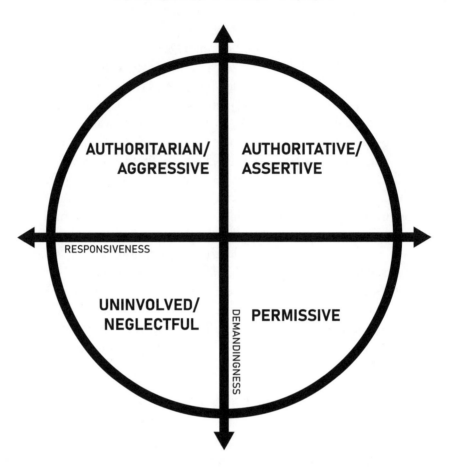

Most parenting occurs along continuums of responsiveness and demandingness. While most parents don't want to be seen as demanding, setting healthy expectations and boundaries/consequences for when those expectations aren't met is part of the job. Put your initials within whichever quadrant feels most true to the way you parent. Then, reflecting on your own childhood, place an M in whichever quadrant would best describe your mom's parenting and place a D in whichever quadrant would best describe your dad's parenting.

FIGURE 8.12. Parenting Styles Grid.

"pushovers" or "doormats" (some other parent-generated labels for permissive). To this end, it is helpful to have parents begin using these dimensions in relationship to others before they apply them to themselves. Many parents are able to use this language to reflect on their family of origin, identifying their own parents along this continuum. We take our first casual look at this during intake. In our assessment forms, we include a section that asks about current parenting practices and hones in on how much discipline the parents believe the identified client needs and how they currently provide that discipline. At that time, I usually explain, "Within a parenting partnership, there is usually one parent who is more permissive and one parent who is more authoritarian" and ask how they would describe their parenting partnership. Since this is our first meeting and we are still in an information-gathering stage of therapy while also building initial rapport, I simply jot down the gist of however the parents respond, knowing that we will come back to the matter later on.

Sometimes it might be easier to talk with parents about what they value most in family life. Some parents value rules and rule following, as this provides a structure that keeps everyone safe and helps things run smoothly. Other parents value relationship and intimacy most and may see rule enforcement as a barrier to connection. Still others may value "doing the hard thing anyway"—an expression we use frequently at Nurture House above all else—so homework, chores, and the like must be done before any playtime or connection can occur. These conversations can help ease the way into an exploration of the Parenting Pendulum, helping parents reflect on where they land along a continuum of parenting responses (see Figure 8.13). We like using Newton's Cradle because we believe in the power of the prop to get parents kinesthetically involved and help them anchor the psychoeducation and reflective work more permanently.

The Nuance of "No"

There are those who believe that telling a child "no" can create toxic shame and shut down learning. I think that how the "no" is said, why the "no" is said, and what else is offered in its place can make all the difference in a child's learning and development. When a "no" is given, it should always be clearly articulated by the parent and matched to the developmental need of the child at the particular time that a limit is being set. The age-old parenting response "because I said so" may still be relevant in some situations, but does not afford room for learning and overall development if used too frequently. So then, what are we to do? At Nurture House, we teach parents the three-pronged approach to limit setting developed by the TraumaPlay Institute. TraumaPlay, a flexibly sequential play therapy approach for treating traumatized children, has as one of its core values the importance of *following the child's need* during therapy. This same mantra applies when parents have to set or enforce limits. When a child has broken a limit, the first question needs to be "What sort of discipline is needed here?" I am deeply guided by Vygotsky's work and his zone of proximal development. The word *discipline* comes from the Latin word *disciplina* that means "instruction and training." The root word *discere* means "to learn." TraumaPlay therapists believe that correction is most helpful when it furthers at least one of the developmental processes of childhood. Most parents would agree that there are moments of intense danger when a child must obey right away. When a child is about to run into the street after a ball and the parent yells "Stop!," we all hope that the child does so. However, this form of discipline is only needed in moments of extreme urgency. Helping children grow into the unique adults they are meant to be is much like nurturing the development of a tree from a sapling. We want their roots to grow deep, and we want to plant them in the best soil for optimal development. To this end, we work with parents around a graphic that shows the three needs a child may be expressing in a moment when discipline is required (see Figure 8.14 later in the chapter).

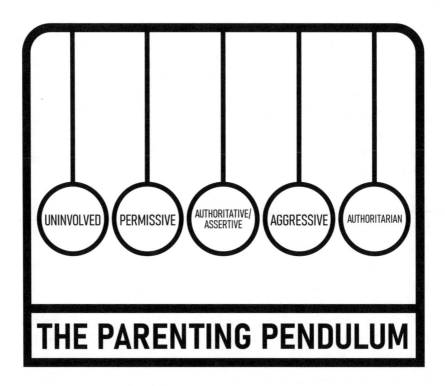

FIGURE 8.13. The Parenting Pendulum.

The "Maybe" Pitfall

One pitfall made by many parents is not saying "no" clearly enough. In fact, perhaps the more dangerous word when it comes to answering the question of dysregulated children is "maybe." Many of the children we see in therapy have anxiety issues, rigid thinking, and obsessive tendencies. Many of them also need a great deal of structure. Parents may believe they are being reasonable, even friendly, by saying "maybe" when their child asks if he can go to the movies later on that day. This vague response that leaves the door open to the possibility of going to the movies later is actually likely to trigger a perseverative response in our anxious clients. The boy here may handle this by cycling the question over and over again internally, hyperfocusing on the possible outing in a way that prohibits him from focusing on schoolwork, chores, or even playtime with friends. The alternative response is that he continues demanding a clear answer, asking his parents over and over again or actively attempting to negotiate while each parent is trying to get other things accomplished. Parents might respond to these repeated intrusions with exasperation, and it is not unusual for the end result of a "maybe" given by a parent early in the day to become a "Well, since you weren't able to wait patiently" or "Because you keep nagging me about it" . . . here it comes . . . the answer is "no." The problem is that at this point the parent is likely frustrated and saying "no" in a sharp, no-nonsense tone potentially aimed at punishing the child for all the extra effort the parent has expended on the issue. However, this is most frequently a parenting mistake. Parental ambivalence, or a hesitancy to be "the bad guy" has encouraged the parent to collude with the most hopeful fantasies of the child who is asking, when the most loving, Safe Boss thing to do would be to bring clarity to the situation. So, for the child and teen clients who need clear answers, the parenting response to a question brings the most peace when it is "yes," "no," or "once x, y, and z have been accomplished."

Giving "Yes"

When a parent gives a "yes," it can go a long way toward putting trust in the tank with a child, especially when that child had early neglect or maltreatment. Trust-Based Relational Intervention, a model developed down at Texas Christian University's Child Development Center, touts itself as a way of giving a "yes" (Purvis, Cross, Dansereau, & Parris, 2013). Daniel Siegel, in his book *The Yes Brain* (Siegel & Bryson, 2018), talks about the scientific data that support the neurobiological pleasure surges that we experience when we are given a "yes." I don't want to offer any strategy as a parent that I wouldn't be willing to try myself, so when I was first learning about giving "yes," I made it my primary parenting focus for the week. What I came to understand is that I am much more likely to say "no," "not now," "maybe later," and other negative responses simply because it is easier and requires less energy than coming up with a creative way to give at least a partial "yes," especially when my mind is deeply involved in something else.

Tonya, a little girl adopted from India, taught me the most about the importance of giving "yes." She was adopted at age 2; her parents showed up at the orphanage unannounced. This particular orphanage had a policy of not permitting potential adoptive parents to venture beyond the main welcome room, but on this particular day, all the care workers were occupied with meal time. The parents walked in on at least a dozen young children scrambling for handfuls of the bucket of rice that had just been poured directly onto the cement floor. Once such a child is home in America, the stakes for giving "yes" and putting trust in the tank are much higher than they are for a securely attached child who has had no food insecurities. Sometimes the insecurity or anxiety that is triggered by a "no" around food can be due to neglect or maltreatment, as in the case above. With other clients, their metabolism may be revved up to such an extent that they simply need to eat more frequently. Some children have a heightened internal sensitivity or interoception around hunger. When they are hungry, it becomes a full-body experience for them. So, how and when we give "yes" can be highly child-dependent, contextualized by a parent's understanding of their child's Window of Tolerance for distress specific to food issues. Let's say that I'm in the middle of making dinner, and it will be ready at 5:30. My son (whose Window of Tolerance for delaying gratification is pretty wide) comes running in from playing outside at 5 o'clock and asks, "Mom, can I have a granola bar?" Because there has been no food insecurity and because our bond is secure, he will accept a "no" easily, give me a quick squeeze, and run off to play for another half-hour.

The child who was clawing her way to food on the middle of the orphanage floor will not be able to accept the "no." One of the core questions for this child is "Will there be enough for me?" If I give a hard "no" to the granola bar, I am likely to feed her fear-based brain and trigger a full-blown amygdala meltdown. For this child, I am going to squat down next to her and make loving eye contact, saying, "Thanks for using your good words to let me know what you want." Beyond this immediate response, there are several alternatives. The truth is that I never make food the hill to die on for children who come from hard places. However, as therapists, our job is to understand what the family system can hold and work within these parameters. Some of the parents I work with have such high control needs, or such strong beliefs about healthy eating, that they simply cannot let a child have a snack half an hour before dinner time. We can still help these parents give a partial "yes." After delighting in the child for using her voice to ask, the parent can say, "Let's go together to the pantry and pick one out. Do you want an apple bar or a chocolate chip bar?" The child chooses. "Do you want to keep it in your pocket until you've eaten your green beans or put it right next to your plate?" Offering these sets of choices is a variation of the "yes" that may help mitigate the child's perceived need, stretching the Window of Tolerance enough to make it through the next half-hour. One of the important distinctions in this response pattern is that the parent sticks together with the child while getting the granola bar and deciding what to do with it. Especially for children with complex trauma, pairing *relationship with resource* becomes an important treatment goal. It is part of what we find so powerful about developing a Nurture Nook for parent and child. Laughter, nurture, and need meeting all take place in the Nurture Nook in combination with the parent.

Are Boundaries Really Necessary?

Yes. Children need boundaries like they need water. In play therapy, the child's neuroception of safety can be compromised when the therapist is anxious about setting boundaries. The therapist's decision-making process often remains internal and can move the clinician's focus from being wholly present for the client to a self-focused dialogue (i.e., "Oh boy, he's about to dump a bunch of sand out of the sand tray. . . . Should I allow that, or limit it, or redirect? I should know the answer to this by now. What's wrong with me? Maybe I'm being too controlling?"). During this internal monologue, the child may feel adrift in the playroom, not fully anchored by his safe grown-up. One of the roles of a clinical supervisor is helping new clinicians articulate their boundaries and then practice setting them. We often do this playfully in role-play scenarios during live supervision. Such a process is equally applicable to parent training. Parents may not have reflected deeply on their own boundaries until the child has pushed them, or, in some cases, run right over them. When parents are spending enormous amounts of internal energy trying to decide if a boundary needs to be set, they are not fully present for the child. So, we work together, therapist and each parent, to uncover the parent's established boundaries and those that are under construction. Sometimes a parent's boundaries are more rigid than they need to be. This can usually be traced back to a core anxiety, a fear of being out of control, or the way that person was parented. It is part of the attuned therapist's job to help each parent reflect on these boundaries, to be curious about what would happen if the parent became less rigid in an area, and to practice letting go. Other parents have almost no boundaries, and an attuned therapist helps them develop appropriate boundaries where none exist. When we don't set boundaries, we end up feeling resentful (Brown, 2015).

Our worst parenting moments are often when we have been giving and giving and giving. When our child asks for one more thing or violates one more boundary, we explode with resentment, calling our children spoiled, entitled, or just plain selfish. This reminds me of a quote by blogger and author Rachel Wolchin, "Givers need to set limits because takers never do." Although it may not be PC to say so, children are takers. They will take as much time, attention, energy, and resources as we give them and come back asking for more. That's OK. It's even developmentally appropriate, and they certainly do give back in their own ways. Therapists can help parents protect themselves and their children from the overflow of unchecked resentment. This begins with clarifying boundaries. The Brene Brown mantra, taken from *Dare to Lead,* is "Clear is Kind. Unclear is Unkind." I share this with parents often and sometimes hear them chanting it as we are practicing the specific boundary-setting work needed for their child.

Boundary Work

In TraumaPlay, we engage in boundaries work with parents on three levels:

1. We set our own boundaries clearly and enforce them calmly, and with warmth in our relationships with both the child or teen client and the parents, we are clear but kind.
2. We provide a safe space for the parent to reflect on their boundaries (this may include family of origin work that requires vulnerability, receiving some psychoeducation in titrated doses that can be digested, and receiving permission when needed to set boundaries more effectively).
3. We do *in vivo* role-plays in which we, the clinicians, become the child, while the parent practices new skills.

When we are doing *in vivo* role-plays with supervisees or parents, we ask them to create a signal for when or if they need a time-out. This serves two useful purposes. The first goal is to help parents start to recognize the somatic sensations of being swamped or overwhelmed and give an external cue that they are present. Helping parents learn to mindfully notice their neurophysiological reactions to the stress of having a boundary violated is the first step in helping them set boundaries differently. Parents may also have a core cognitive distortion insisting that they are helpless to do anything about this boundary violation. Such entrenched cognitions will show up with somatic markers, too, and helping parents become aware of what their bodies are telling them. This can be the beginning of their recognizing that a boundary needs to be set. Once you, the therapist, have developed a good rapport and safety with the parents, the parent can try out new behaviors. You become the secure base for the parent to explore new patterns of responding.

The second goal of giving a signal to step out of the role-play is to slow everything down and invite the parent to bring their Choosing Mind to bear on the boundary issue at hand. Imagine that I, while playing the impulsive 8-year-old daughter of a dad who has struggled with passivity in his parenting, pick up a handful of sand and gesture as if I am going to throw it in his face. Most parents would experience this in their sympathetic nervous system as a potential threat; they might raise their voice, yelling "Stop!," in response. When the dad experiences one of these parasympathetic surges start to occur within his body, he holds up the time-out signal. We laugh together, as laughter is a great release of pent-up anxiety, acknowledge that this is a behavior the dad feels requires a boundary, and then craft the language of the limit and the alternatives together. We subsequently re-invest in the role-play and process what it felt like for the parent to give this newly crafted response. Most parents don't love role-play, and many will actively try to avoid it, *but parent coaching is most effective when the physiology becomes engaged,* not just the cognitive process of receiving information. Parents are literally learning to regulate their way through limit setting when they role-play with us in real time. Moreover, playing the role of a child in a live role-play with a parent is one of the few times when therapists get to act truly childish!

Danny Silk, in his parent coaching workshops, asks parents to create an internal image of their own garden—including what plants they might like to grow there, what kind of gate they would want the space to have, where the walking paths and sitting spots would be located. Would there be any water in your garden? He then compares the child without boundaries to a large animal barreling into the garden, destroying the edges of the flower beds, muddying the paths, and so on. He goes on to encourage parents to create an internal visual image of maintaining the boundaries of their happy garden when they say "no" to interactions or requests that would destroy it. How does one do this? Well, the problem the child is trying to foist onto the parent needs to become a possible problem for the child.

Silk gives an example of a teenager who leaves her backpack on the school bus. The first time this happens, the teenager comes home and, when it is time to do her homework, realizes she has left her bag on the bus. The mom exclaims, "This is the second time this week! You are so irresponsible! Do you know how much it will put off dinner for me to drive all the way back to the school to get it for you? Honestly, you never think of anyone but yourself!" This tirade continues all the way back to the school, while the teenager tunes it out. This teenager has learned that although her mother will grump and complain, if she weathers the storm of her mom's anger, she will still get the outcome she needs without having to do anything differently (or difficult) herself. It's only a problem for Mom each time, and nothing in the system is changing. How do we make it a possible problem for the teen? The next time her daughter leaves her backpack on the bus and then comes running for assistance, saying, "I have a quiz tomorrow and all my notes are in my backpack! I need to get it!," Mom matches her concern with this: "Oh no! You told me last night that this quiz equals half your grade . . . and you left your backpack on the bus. That stinks! What are you going to do?" The teenage daughter is likely to be caught off-guard, thinking, *What do you mean, what am I going to do about it? You are usually the one who does something about it.* "Well, can you take me back to school to get it? I really need it." Mom would then respond, "Gosh, it's a real problem for you, and I would like to help. You can ask a friend to come get you and take you back (which might save you some money)." Or, "I am happy to let you use my Uber app and see how much a ride would cost." Or, "You can pay me to take you. . . . I'll take 10% off whatever Uber would charge because I love you, or I can take you to school a little early if you decide it's not worth going back to get it tonight. Let me know what you decide. I'm gonna go start dinner." This is the beginning of making the repeated error a *possible problem for her daughter*. If she fails the quiz because she hasn't made it a priority to bring the notes home, that, too, will be good learning experience for her.

The Three Roots of Discipline

Safety and the No-Go Limit

Sometimes the first and only need in a moment of discipline is to provide safety. This safety may reference the child's interaction with the immediate environment (as when a child is about to stick a fork into an electric socket). This safety might extend to other siblings or adults in the home (the child is limited from hitting his sister in frustration). This safety might also extend to the rest of the community (the teenager is not allowed to blast his music on the front porch if others nearby are enjoying a quiet evening on their front porches). When the identified need is to provide a clear limit that must be quickly enforced, we ask parents to limit the object or the use of the object, while providing a couple of alternatives for its use. This limit-setting model was created by Garry Landreth (2002) and has been absorbed and practiced by generations of play therapists. It is not always intuitive or easy to learn this model, and parents need support in absorbing it. Recently, a supervisee had a child uncap a Sharpie and move toward her face, saying, "I'm gonna draw a mustache on you!" She reacted quickly, because we'd been practicing in supervision, and was able to say, "Oh! You really want to Sharpie me, but I am not for Sharpying. You can Sharpie on the paper or on the cardboard." The child who is hammering in the garage while Dad is working on the car pulls back the hammer to wack a porcelain plate. The grown-up says, "The hammer is not for using on the plate. You can use the hammer on the wood or on the ground." Limiting the use of an object is less likely to be internalized by the child as a sense of their own badness, but rather will lead to an internalized structure and potential for self-control.

When Children Need to Learn Something New or Practice More

The second root underlying a discipline moment is a child's need to learn something new or practice something more frequently. In these cases, a "redo" is the most effective discipline strategy. When a child is being demanding, insisting, "Give me milk!," the wise parent is one who has the child redo the request with "asking" words. When a child barges into a room without knocking, a wise parent says, "You're still learning to knock before you open the door. Let's go back and redo that." This allows the child to practice. Remember that one of our goals as clinicians is to help parents provide opportunities for clients to lay down new neural pathways and deepen existing pathways. This requires practice, practice, and more practice. The other positive aspect of a redo is that it, too, does not assign badness to the child, but simply reminds both parent and child that learning and practice are still required for a particular skill. Perhaps the child suddenly grabs a toy from his brother. The need-knowing parent will have that child redo the interaction with his brother, giving the toy back to the brother and coaching the child to ask for it instead of grabbing it. This strategy is, at first glance, not difficult. However, when you have repeated the same redo lots and lots of times, parents can begin to feel like they are hitting their heads against a brick wall. This is when the role of the therapist moves into that of cheerleader and a reminder of the way that neurobiological wiring occurs.

Negotiate Getting Needs Met

Lastly, in some cases, the most important need for the child is for the child to negotiate getting her needs met. This strategy can be particularly important for children who come from trauma, neglect, or have had multiple caregiver disruptions. These children did not have people around who were meeting their needs regularly, so they developed a control foundation versus a trust foundation. For these children, recognizing that one person in the relationship wants one thing and that they want another—and that negotiation can result in a compromise where one person gets some of what she needs and the other person gets some of what he needs—is the most important way to grow trust and relationship. Truly, beyond the parent–child relationship, I have trouble thinking of any healthy relationships in which one person obeys the other person right away and without question, without any discourse, compromise, negotiation, or listening to alternate points of view. Although compromise is often the hardest of the three types of discipline to provide, because it requires additional time and, in all honesty, more mental energy from the grown-up to help structure the compromises, it is the most likely to result in healthy adults who can negotiate getting their needs met in a variety of settings. The tree featured in Figure 8.14 reminds parents of these three root needs associated with discipline and shows the branches of the tree that are developed through setting limits with alternatives and asking for compromises, while keeping the redo as the central strategy for growth. Redos come in many shapes and sizes. At Nurture House, we probably engage in 50 redos a day as a team, but this pairing of the physical reenactment (walking instead of running, holding out a hand while asking for a toy from a peer) with kind words (asking instead of telling) is the bedrock strategy for laying down new neural wiring. To this end, we have developed "The Three Roots of Discipline" handout (see Figure 8.14) that can serve as a decision-making tree for how to respond when a child is in need of direction or correction.

THE THREE ROOTS OF DISCIPLINE

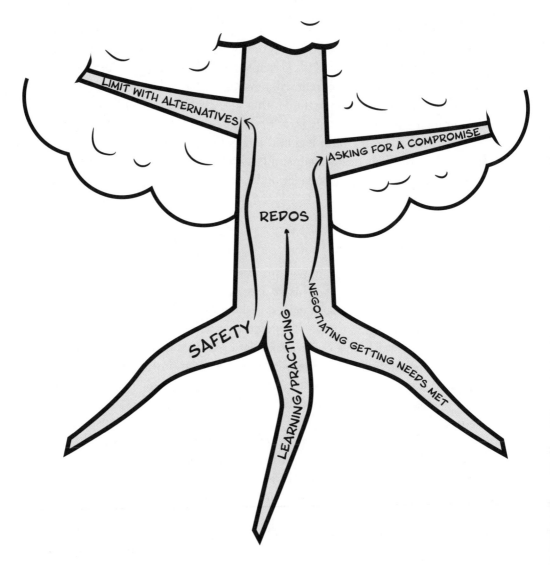

FIGURE 8.14. The Three Roots of Discipline.

Take Two

This adaptation of the redo allows for both parents and children to make slight shifts in their responses as a scenario is replayed. We have physical Take Two clapboards at Nurture House, and I would encourage the addition of this 3-D play tool for therapists who are helping parents and children try to learn with a redo. One of my favorite parts of the Take Two intervention is that it encourages parents to take responsibility for any part of their own communication that may need to be tried again . . . perhaps they used unkind words, perhaps they used a harsh tone of voice, perhaps they forgot to give their child time to respond before they escalated. This provides good learning for the parent, good modeling for the child, and a corrective emotional experience for both as they redo the scene according to the Take Two board. The handout in Figure 8.15 gives room for the parent to briefly describe the

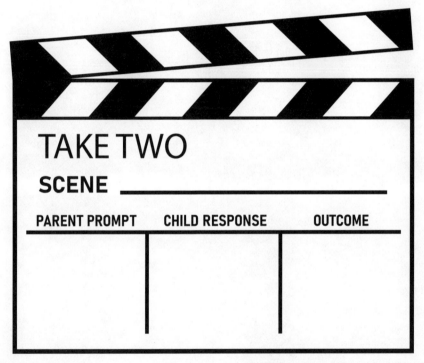

Scene: Name the event.

Parent Prompt: Write in the short phrase you used to help your child practice communicating differently.

Child Response: What the child said or did.

Outcome: How did it end the second time?

FIGURE 8.15. Take Two Handout.

behavior that was inappropriate, then to record the parenting prompt they gave for a redo, the child's response, and the outcome. For example, a child might demand milk from his father, demanding, "I WANT MILK!" His dad would give the prompt "I need you to ask me nicely." The child's response would then be "May I have milk, please?"; the outcome that the child got to have his glass of milk. A second hand-out (see Figure 8.16), offering six blank Take Twos, is included so that parents can practice the Take Two intervention in lots of situations at home, record them, and bring them back to the next session for processing.

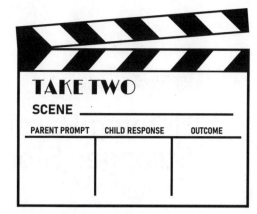

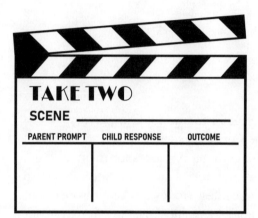

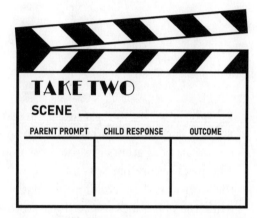

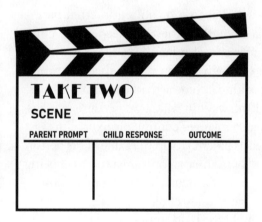

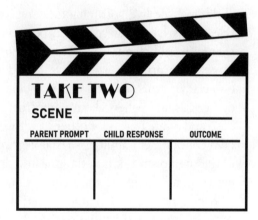

FIGURE 8.16. Take Two Parent Homework.

CHAPTER 9

Helping Parents Become Stronger Storykeepers

S tories are the way we understand ourselves in the world. Our parents are the first ones to tell stories about us, and the stories they tell shape our personhood for a lifetime. Parents are the most powerful early Storykeepers for their children. The word *history* has within it the words *his* and *story*. Parents are meant to keep the stories of their children, as many of the earliest stories are being worked out while the child does not yet have words or autobiographical memory to narrate for himself. While children so desperately need this storykeeping capacity, it requires that parents have fairly coherent narratives of their own stories. But, many of the children I see live with chaotic caregivers who have no organized internal narrative themselves. Our goal then becomes to strengthen the Storykeeper. We child therapists embrace a Cascade of Care in our work with families and begin from a place of ensuring that we have first done our own person of the therapist work, especially as this self-exploration includes looking at our own attachment histories, our values and beliefs about parenting, and the ways in which we become a secure base and a safe haven for others. Our work also involves continually expanding our own containment abilities so that we can teach parents to do the same. This person of the therapist work is not a "one and done," but rather an ongoing process of being curious and compassionate about ourselves and particularly about our responses to triggering family dynamics in our work. TraumaPlay clinicians work on making sense of their own histories so that they can hold the hard stories of the parents and children in their care. You have already read about how we hold the story of the parent's early history in order to help her experience having her story held and shared by another without judgment (Chapter 3). This chapter will give multiple examples of practical play-based strategies that clinicians can use to facilitate coherence in parent–child–family narratives. While co-created story is always therapeutic and strengthens connections among family members, it is especially important when the child has existed in a vacuum of information, filled in unknown details with misinformation, or needs to have his cognitive distortions changed and attachments enhanced. This chapter will give examples of such work happening in the sand tray, in art, in verbal storytelling form, and, of course, in play. Song, poetry, visual media, and other mediums allow for an ever-expanding use of expressive mediums to help children and their caregivers approach hard things. Expressive therapies encourage clients to approach content in the way that most readily captures their right-brain knowledge and pairs it together with their left-brain narrative (Graves-Alcorn & Green, 2014; Graves-Alcorn & Kagin, 2017; Landgarten, 1987; Lowenfeld, 1950; Malchiodi, 2013, 2020; Rose, 2017; Salters, 2013).

The Marschak Interaction Method (MIM) offers a prompt for parents that instructs them to *Tell a story about when your child was a baby, beginning with "When you were a little baby. . . ."* We have incorporated this prompt into our Nurture House Dyadic Assessment (NHDA) and heard thousands of baby stories. The clinical presentations can vary immensely. Clearly, these stories speak to the earliest impressions of how the child's arrival affected the parent. Particularly with foster and adoptive families, but in many biologically intact families (especially when postpartum depression, medical trauma in the child's earliest years, or other extreme stressors may have interrupted the attachment relationship), we incorporate storytelling aimed at amplifying the nurture, competency, and regulation in the relationship. We call these Delighting-In Stories and they are normally told by the parent to the therapist while the child is snuggling with the parent, enjoying a shared snack, at either the beginning or the end of session (see Chapter 6). What we have learned the hard way over the years is that not every parent is skilled in telling a story with a beginning, a middle, and an end or at telling a story that celebrates the child or the parent–child relationship in some way. To this end, we have developed a set of Delighting-In Story Starters for parents. We go over these in a parent coaching session, perhaps helping parents create and/or rehearse the first few that will be told and supporting them through the process. This template helps parents become comfortable with the mechanisms of storytelling as they apply to the therapeutic milieu so that when it comes time to narrate the harder stories of the family, they can focus their whole energy on the content and delivery and not have to worry about the story structure.

Nurturing Narration

Recently, as I was writing about the triune brain, my fingers tripped over the keys, and I misspelled the word *neocortex,* somehow adding a "t" at the end. Just before I pressed the backspace key, I read the new word, *neocortext,* and I thought, "yes!" It struck me that this new word might be the perfect expression for the coherent narrative building we are trying to influence in the families with whom we work. *Neo-* ("new"), *cor-* (the "core" or "essence"), *text* ("story") . . . put it all together and you have a word that means the "new core story." Isn't this one of the goals of reworking trauma? We hope for the final encoding of a trauma story to acknowledge the hurt, injustice, or sudden loss, but to have the emotional toxicity leached from it, while the survivor's strengths are woven throughout. A new encoding of the essence of the story often includes parent-assisted cognitive interweaves (PACIs) and is one of the most important jobs a therapist can facilitate in helping parents become partners in their child's healing process. Additionally, emotional literacy includes having your emotions held by someone else (Panksepp, 1998; Panksepp & Biven, 2012). So, what we will dig into in this chapter is how we take bits and pieces of a narrative, and develop a neocortext that can invite the linear narrative, the cognitions, emotions, and somatic experiences that are to be shared by the parent and child, or—even better—by the whole family system.

There is an old Hopi proverb: "Those who tell the stories rule the world." Parents are the Storykeepers for their children, and in no small part this means that the stories parents tell rule the stories that children tell to themselves. Stories shape our sense of self even before we have autobiographical memory. I have clients who regularly tell me a story about their infancy or toddler years, but only "remember" the story because it has been told to them over and over again. The power of the parental voice in shaping our stories about ourselves and the world are part of what can lay the groundwork for parental alienation syndrome (PAS) in divorcing families or set the stage for a legacy of warm memories of family.

Given the power of stories in shaping children's sense of themselves and the world, it is good for parents to be careful, thoughtful, and intentional about the stories they tell and how and when they tell them. One might think that this comes intuitively, but there are many parents who have difficulty with appropriate storytelling. Some parents read the task out loud and then lean their bodies in toward their child with delight or pick the child up and pull the child onto their laps, and tell a story about how cute and snuggly they were, what the child's first words were, how excited everyone was to meet the new baby. Other parents will read the task and say, "When you were a little baby . . ." and a long pause ensues. Then one of the parents may say "You were so fat!" or "You cried all the time" or "You didn't sleep through the night for a year." The most difficult story that I have listened to was told by a dad who was heavy into fitness. His story went like this: "When you were a baby, I would put you in the jog stroller to try to go for a run in the morning. But your arms were so fat, they would fall out of the stroller and get caught in the spokes, and I would have to stop and put your arms back in the stroller. I don't think I got a good work-out the whole first year you were alive!" Some stories have been shocking and some have made me smile all over. Some parents were so overwhelmed by stress or preoccupied when their children were babies that they have difficulty remembering any specific details to package in a story. Other parents remember only the hardest parts of the child's earliest life, offering a story like the following: "When you were a little baby, you cried all the time. You didn't like the formula that we gave you, and you wouldn't go to sleep. Mommy and Daddy were up all night with you!"

One exceptional story went like this. Mom reads the task out loud, gets a big smile on her face, and looks in her daughter's eyes while saying, in a tone infused with delight, "When you were a little baby, I used to dress you up in cute little outfits and sometimes little baby sunglasses, and I would put you in the stroller, and we would go out strolling." The daughter interrupts and makes the baby sign gesture for milk while saying, "And sometimes I did sign language." Mom replied, while making the same sign, "You did, you did sign language and what did that mean? What would you tell me?" Her daughter says, "Milk." Mom replies, "Yes, you wanted milk 'cause you were thirsty. And we would stroll around and we'd stop and have some milk, and we might stop to pet a dog, and then after awhile, I would look at my watch and I would say, 'It's almost time for Daddy to come home, we better go home,'" and you would say, 'goo goo, gaa, gaa,' and I would take you home." Clearly, the little girl knew some of the details of this story already, so it may have been shared before. Mom's story had a clear beginning, a middle, and an end. It gave details of Mom's caretaking, her daughter's ability to use her voice to ask for what she needed, and Mom's pattern of meeting a need when her daughter would ask. This kind of story translates Mom's core text about her experience of her daughter in early childhood for her daughter in a way that supports the following core text for her child. "I am . . . delightful. I am . . . able to ask for what I need. I am . . . seen." Powerful I am's for this little girl.

A clear, coherent story is one that has a beginning, a middle, and an end. Especially when children have experienced any of the adverse childhood experiences (ACEs; Anda et al., 2006; Dube et al., 2003; Felitti et al., 1998), it is one of the jobs of the Safe Boss to help bring coherence to their narrative regarding those events. The times when a child most needs coherence, however, is when he is often least likely to get it. I had this truth brought home to me when I mistakenly tried to do timeline work with a dyad before the dad had brought enough coherence to his own story. Edward was a 35-year-old who had developed a drug addiction early on in his marriage. He and his wife divorced and his two children, both preschoolers at the time, lived with his former wife and saw him intermittently. He eventually got into a rehab program, spent several months in treatment, and worked his way back to supervised visits with his children. He was working his program and wanted a renewed relationship with his kids more than anything. I had been seeing his daughter for some time and was the natural choice to supervise therapeutic visitations. We began with several sessions of playful, low-stress getting to know you (again) activities. I trained him on how to follow his daughter's lead in play as well, and she enjoyed playing with him. I had collateral sessions with Dad, preparing him to be a bigger, stronger, wiser, kind container. We practiced reflecting and holding his daughter's big feelings (I played the daughter in these role-plays), and I got the details that he could recollect about the events leading up to his addiction. Eventually, I felt that they were both ready to do timeline work. I taped together several pieces of construction paper, glued a long ribbon down its center, and asked the daughter to tell me the story of her early life when Dad was still at home—one he might not remember. What follows is a transcribed record of the session with some details changed to protect the family's anonymity:

DAD: Her crib was filled with teddy bears. . . .

DAUGHTER: I also had bunnies!

DAD: And she wanted to sleep with them.

PARIS: Really!

DAD: Sleep with all those stuffed animals. Not a blankie or cuddly loveys, but all her bears.

PARIS: Do you remember that?

DAUGHTER: Uh, huh. It was funny! (*refocusing on the timeline*) Then Mom and Dad were divorced . . . you divorced when . . .

DAD: Were we divorced when you were 5? How old am I now?

DAUGHTER: You are 35.

DAD: (*scrunching up his face in thought*) So, we've been divorced 4 years.

DAUGHTER: I was 4. (*Silence.*) What grade was I in? That was when I started playing . . . no. I started playing soccer when I was . . . (*Runs her fingers through her hair while she stares at the timeline with the marker in her other hand.*)

DAD: (*after a pause, looking at the therapist and smiling apologetically*) We're having a hard time with this timeline. I think we're both having a hard time coming up with . . .

PARIS: (*reassuringly*) So, she was 4 when you got divorced.

DAUGHTER: (*After writing that down, drops the pen on the table.*) You can go now, Dad.

[While Dad picks up the pen, I engage the client around a memory of his own.]

PARIS: What do you remember about that time?

DAUGHTER: Um. We all got together at my old house and sat down on the crouton thing. . . .

DAD: Futon . . . (*They both laugh.*)

PARIS: (*laughing with them*) The crouton futon [which becomes a running joke for them].

DAUGHTER: Then they said that they were getting divorced, but I didn't know what that means. And they told me that they weren't going to live with each other anymore. Then my Dad started living with my grandparents.

PARIS: So, at that point you stayed in the house you'd been living in?

DAUGHTER: Mmhmm. And like every weekend, we stayed with our dad.

PARIS: Did you move in with Mom before or after Dad started doing drugs?

DAUGHTER: (*with assurance*) After.

PARIS: What do you remember about that?

DAUGHTER: (*staring out the window*) The first time . . . he wouldn't wake up. I remember when he wouldn't wake up then. . . . I don't remember anything else but that first time when he didn't wake up.

PARIS: We should probably put that on the timeline, 'cause that's something you've talked about a lot, him sleeping . . . or not waking up.

DAD: (*with the marker in his hand*) So . . . , Dad didn't wake up one morning. (*speaking out loud slowly as he writes*) Dad . . . didn't . . . wake . . . up . . . one . . .

DAUGHTER: Dad didn't wake up a lot of mornings.

DAD: (*to his credit, nodding as a way to say he hears her, also repeats*) Dad didn't wake up a lot of mornings.

[There it is right there, the holding of the story.]

PARIS: And you noticed that this was a big change from how he had been. And what did you start thinking at that point?

DAUGHTER: Worried.

DAD: That's when I went to Colorado. I was inpatient for 2 months.

PARIS: I remember you guys saying that Dad was in Colorado. Did you go there to see him?

DAUGHTER: (*participating more eagerly now*) Yeah, once.

PARIS: When did he come back?

DAUGHTER: It was about a year ago now?

PARIS: Then you felt like Dad was really home and was really trying to work on things?

DAUGHTER: He painted his house.

PARIS: Was that a big deal?

DAD: I painted the playroom.

PARIS: What color did you paint it?

[Dad starts to respond, but his daughter interrupts with "He painted it like . . . like . . . that out there . . . (*gesturing to the blue sky outside the window*). A blue sky! He had blue around the walls, a sun, trees, and he made the house yellow and red."]

PARIS: You remember in great detail what he painted. Sounds like that was important to you, that he had spent some time fixing up his house for you.

Dad and daughter were both smiling from ear to ear. Although it was difficult to process the yucky stuff, coming out on the other side on the timeline provided a shared sense of accomplishment for both. Dad beamed ear to ear as he listened to his daughter rehearse the proof that he was back to stay—the details of the mural in their bonus room. Whenever possible, when doing timeline work with regard to a trauma in the family system that involves disruption, beginning from a place of safe connection before the trauma occurred (in this case, two traumas: addiction and divorce); processing through the hardest parts, naming them in shared space on the timeline; and ending up in a place where a connection has been restored are optimal. The other learning for me, from this session, was that it is helpful to more fully support the parent in establishing coherence in their own narrative of events before co-creating a narrative with the child. This daughter provided more structuring at the beginning of the session than we would like to see. Adequate preparation for dyadic timeline work will sometimes require additional collateral sessions focused on concretizing the parent's timeline/story work before doing timeline work with both parent and child together.

The We Are's

As we reflect on the stories parents tell during the NHDA that begin with the prompt "When you were a little baby . . ." we find a second set of core texts that arise from stories like these. I call them the "We are's." When the dad tells his son about how he was so fat, dad had to stop the jog stroller over and over again when he really wanted to exercise, this dyad may develop a shared core text that sounds like this: "We are constantly having to negotiate what I want (dad) with what you need (son)." In the story mom tells about their daily walks in the neighborhood, a mom and her daughter may develop a shared core text that sounds like this: "We are a great team. We are exploring and enjoying the world together. We are living within predictable routines." Core cognitions that guide the dyadic dance between parent and child can be heard as we listen for the "We are's." The dad–son story may yield the belief "We can get back on track after we take care of your need." The mom–daughter story may yield the belief "We can explore the world together." When the pair stops to pet a dog, this also might yield the belief "We can experience new things together."

After listening to (and watching) thousands of stories, I am more certain than ever that many parents need support in learning to create and deliver stories that support positive I am's for the child and We are's for the dyad. Intergenerational trauma, negative self-talk scripts, stress in the system, and a lack of having been told loving stories themselves keep parents stuck in unhealthy storytelling patterns. At Nurture House, at some point in attachment-enhancement sessions, the parent is asked to tell a Delighting-In Story: a story that rehearses a child's new competency or competency enhancement, a moment of joy, a moment of shared laughter, or a moment of shared novel experience. We have developed a storytelling template that helps to structure parents as they create these Delighting-In Stories. Part of this practice is preparing parents to tell more difficult stories, stories that may encompass traumatic content or moments when a rupture was created between a parent and child.

The second storykeeping tool involves parent reflection and helps the parent focus on the *I am* and *We are* takeaways from the story. To illustrate this tool, I will start with a case example. I have been working with an ambivalently anxious, adopted 9-year-old whom we will call Danny. He is almost as big as his adoptive mother, and he rages "round the clock" according to Mom. When he appears in my lobby, his head is pushed into Mom's chest or armpit. He has a great deal of difficulty transitioning from the lobby to any of our treatment spaces and became almost frozen one day when I entered the lobby to take them back to a space. I offered a choice of two treatment rooms that I knew he preferred, and he whispered something to Mom. Mom, Danny, and I had already been working on helping Danny use his voice to ask for what he wants/needs, so Mom said, "Remember, Danny, you can ask Miss Paris that yourself." I responded, "I am right here to listen, and if it is at all possible, I will try to give you a 'yes.'" I had a feeling that what he wanted to ask was if we could start our session outside in the backyard, as it was the first sunny day in a week. I gave him several opportunities to ask and then invited Mom to stand (and he stood up with her, as he was basically "attached" to her). I said, "It seems really hard for Danny to ask for what he is wanting, so let's get our bodies moving—because sometimes that helps," and Mom and I began shuffling across the room to the snug hallway that separates the sand tray room from the lobby. A small smile began to emerge on Danny's face, and his head came out of Mom's armpit as we all shuffled together. However, once we got into the hallway and were faced with the actual choice between rooms, he sunk back into Mom's shoulder. Mom sat down on the staircase (and the client right along with her); I quickly put the EMDR buzzies in his socks. I switched gears quickly and said, "Mom, it seems like it is too hard just now for Danny to make a decision or to ask for what he needs. Let's just give him a minute, and you and I can talk. Can you tell me a story about one thing you saw Danny do this week that was hard, but that he did because you two were sticking together?" This mantra, captured in Figure 8.10, can be woven into many difficult stories as a hopeful outcome of connection: When we stick together, we can do hard things. This extends past the initial hard moment experienced by the family to the keeping of the story by parent and child together. In these cases, it helps tremendously if the parent is able to revisit the narrative whenever the child needs to revisit it. This revisiting may stem from needing to feel connected to the caregiver; it might stem from needing to clarify a detail or to ask a question, or simply to ensure that the parent is still strong enough to hold the story.

The Third Ear

The power of passive listening is one that parents often have trouble understanding. When children are being talked to, especially about things they have done wrong or about things that were scary, these comments can result in the immediate and unconscious raising of their defenses. Being talked about, instead of being talked to, puts children in a listening posture. However, the talking about is not the kind where two people go and complain about a third party behind that person's back, but where the third person gets to receive the story of what happened without being asked to respond, accept the story, or deny it in any way.

When a child experiences the intensity of her parent's gaze and the potential pressure of having to respond to whatever the parent has said, she is less available to truly hear what the parent is saying. When the child absorbs the story through the power of passive listening, as the parent tells the therapist the story, her defenses go down and the child is more like a sponge, soaking in both the content and the underlying messages. The parent's intensity is being held by the therapist, not by the child. This provides relief from the spotlight and an ability to restfully digest the details. John, a 15-year-old adopted boy, is one such client. He struggles with lots of fears and has recently been diagnosed with obsessive-compulsive disorder. He is finding the psychiatric appointments very scary and is soothed by having Mom narrate their experiences. He will sit in the swing (see Figure 9.1) and request the TheraTappers, and then ask Mom to tell the story of what happened with each of the psychiatrists they visited.

Sometimes parents carry so much of their own pain that they find it difficult to fully meet the child in their anguish. A case example may help illustrate this. A

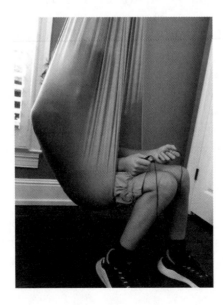

FIGURE 9.1. Listening with the Third Ear.

dad sought out my services after a local court ordered that his 4-year-old son Ricky soon begin visitation with a mother he hadn't seen in at least 2 years. The mother had mental health issues of sudden onset and abruptly disappeared from her child's life, leaving a question mark about whether or not some form of abuse occurred during the periods of her caretaking when Dad had been at work. We decided that the first "Hello" session would happen in the kitchen of Nurture House, that Dad would be present as well, and that we would all bake cookies together. Mom was appropriate and nurturing. Mom and Dad were respectful of one another and therapist-facilitated interactions. Mom came to several more sessions with the client—pushing him on the tire swing in the backyard of Nurture House, creating art with him, hearing about his preschool experiences, and beginning to build some new memories. Then one mid-winter morning, Dad and Ricky waited in the lobby . . . and waited . . . and waited. Mom never came. The intense confusion and sadness experienced by Ricky were palpably felt by both myself and Dad. I will never forget Ricky staring out into the yard through the big picture window in the lobby of Nurture House, saying, "Maybe she didn't come because . . ." Dad and I waited patiently as he searched for words, and he finally said, "because it's cold outside." We did our best to make contact with Mom but were unsuccessful. Then one day, Ricky's dad received a call from the police. Mom had been found in her apartment in a state of both physical and mental decline. She was readmitted to an inpatient program, and the visits with her son were indefinitely discontinued.

The next few sessions involved holding this child's grief and bewilderment at his mother's sudden absence. Dad was also grieving Mom's absence, not for his own sake, but as he understood it to be another loss for his son. One of the hardest jobs for clinicians is creating a holding environment for hurting children that also encourages the parent to hold the hurting child's story even as the parent is hurting. This requires first acknowledging the big feelings of the parent and helping him or her to name them. In this case, the father was devastated at what he perceived to be a second abandonment by Mom. He was also simultaneously relieved, as he experienced some relief from the hypervigilance he had been experiencing during the visits (that feeling of waiting for the other shoe to drop). Finally, he deeply wished, as all good enough parents do, that his son did not have to endure the pain of this maternal loss. I felt the need to create space for Dad and Ricky to hold the story together. For preschool-aged children, their story is often told through play, so I invited Dad and Ricky to play together in session. At Ricky's request, we all climbed the stairs to the Nurture House Nook, the smallest, snuggest space we had available. Ricky had brought with him some toys from home. Almost always, when clients bring a toy from home into the play therapy space, it is meaningful and the wise therapist approaches the addition with curiosity and compassion. Ricky had brought a Darth Vader Lego figure and a medical helicopter that he had created from Legos. Ricky's dad had been trained early on in treatment in the child-centered play skills of filial therapy. He had successfully employed these skills during previous sessions. What follows is the play that Ricky created, along with Dad's responses to it. Darth Vader is fighting with another figure from the sand tray.

RICKY: Darth Vader got hurt!

DAD: Oh, no! He's hurt.

RICKY: He's got to go to the hospital to get better! (*Picks up the helicopter and starts making the noises of the chopper blades. I start to hear the themes here of Mom's earlier hospitalizations.*)

DAD: Oh, good. There's a helicopter to take him.

RICKY: Yep, the copter is coming in for a landing!

DAD: (*clearing away a cushion*) Here's a landing place.

[Ricky lands the helicopter and says, "Quick, we've got to get Darth Vader some help!"

Dad creates a makeshift gurney and says, "OK. We can get him to the hospital. Then he'll be OK!"]

RICKY: Put him inside.

[Dad plays out bringing the gurney over to the helicopter and then puts Darth Vader inside. He says in a playful voice, "OK. You guys are good to take off!"]

RICKY: "Roger that!" (*mimicking the tone of his father's voice*) "There's wind. It's hard to take off."

DAD: They can do it!

[Ricky moves the helicopter high into the air while making chopper blade noises, but his hand begins to wobble and the helicopter starts to tip, Darth Vader falls out of the copter and onto the cushion.]

RICKY: Oh no! Darth Vader got more hurt . . . they lost him!

DAD: Oh! It will be all right. The helicopter will come back and take Darth Vader to get help. He'll be all right.

RICKY: (*making noises of thunder and more helicopter wobbling*) They can't come back for him.

DAD: They'll send more help. He'll be OK.

OK. Indulge me a moment, as I geek out in my most play therapist self. Darth Vader is a wounded figure who had started out with a mission for good and ended up hurting others and turning to the dark side. One might see this child's choice of figure as in some ways representing Mom. There had been hope, in the therapeutic reunification process, that she would return to her ability to parent in a healthy way. The helicopter picks her up to take her to the hospital, but then a storm comes (another metaphoric communication of whatever "sudden" devolution of Mom had kept her from coming to meet him). And despite everyone's best efforts, Darth Vader falls out of the rescue vehicle and is even more extensively injured than before, lost to a world of hurt. I am hearing all of this as Ricky's way to begin building a coherent, albeit metaphoric, narrative of what happened with his mother's attempt at a healthy reunification with him, followed by her sudden and complete absence. Dad, however, is having trouble holding this trauma story. He will feel better if Darth Vader can eventually get the help he needs. Here is a fascinating question: Does Dad's subconscious hear the metaphoric story and defend against his own countertransference, his own guilt at what he perceives as allowing his son to experience Mom again and begin to hope for her healthy involvement in his life (although it was court-ordered regardless, and Dad was simply making the most protective choice he could at the time by attempting therapeutic reunification)? Dad was communicating a continued hope that Darth Vader could be saved, but I think what was needed was for Dad to be a big enough, strong enough, wise enough, and kind enough container for his son's big feelings, for his son's truth, as expressed in the play, that Darth Vader was even more sick/hurt/broken than before and that no amount of rescuing would bring him back to health. It is important to remember that while this may or may not be the whole story or even the end of Ricky's story, it is his attempt to make sense of what has happened.

I spoke with Dad for a few minutes after the session and suggested some of what I unpacked above. It wasn't until later in the day that Dad sent me a communication indicating that as he reflected on their play session together, he was able to understand that Ricky was equating Mom with Darth Vader and needed to have his current truth, that Darth Vader had been lost in a world of hurt—separated from help—and that Ricky needed Dad to hold that hard story. Dad was able to reflect on his own experience and acknowledge that he so much wanted for Mom to end up in a healthy place for Ricky that he was clinging to that story, even when doing so did not help Ricky move to acceptance of his current reality. I continue to be in awe, to this day, of this father's ability to face his own big feelings and grow his capacity to hold his son's hard story.

In another session, weeks after the one described above, I offered Ricky and his dad a large sheet of paper. I drew a very large body to represent Dad and a much smaller body to represent Ricky. I then gave them a set of Band-Aids and asked father and son to identify the current hurts that they each carried (see Figure 9.2). Acknowledging their hurts together strengthened their family narrative.

Marcus Learns to Accept Help

Clinicians can help parents learn that their young children are concrete thinkers and therefore reassured by concrete representations of internal states, such as love and belonging. Another way to help parents grow into this is by talking about the

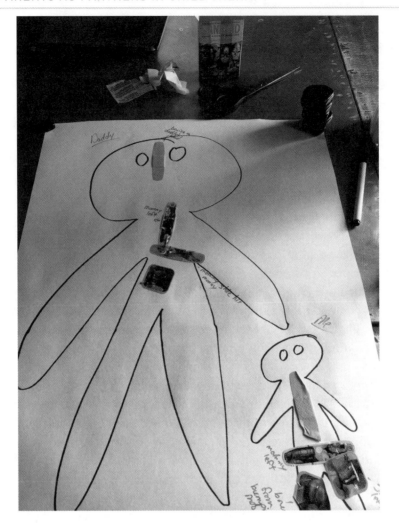

FIGURE 9.2. Parallel Hurts.

power of transitional objects. Little ones are soothed by having a concrete, physical anchor that is associated with the nurture of a parent as they risk separating from that parent to brave other environments (school, church, soccer) on their own. The typical separation anxiety of preschool-aged children can be exponentially magnified in the face of early attachment trauma.

The little boy discussed here, Marcus, was adopted at birth. However, he was born addicted to methamphetamines, which required him to remain in the hospital for over a month, detoxing in ways that are incredibly painful to his body. His adoptive mom detailed her sense of helplessness in the face of his pain. She desperately wanted to comfort him, but he would shake and seize and vomit and sweat and cry inconsolably for hours. Mom touched on her own pain again as she shared these details during our initial session. While her son has no words for this experience, and no autobiographical memories of this period of his life, he has somatic memories that show up in his responses to his parents' current attempts to care for his hurts. He has a great deal of trouble allowing anyone to help him. During one of our first sessions, I employ a boo-boo routine (from the Theraplay model) of checking for hurts. He immediately becomes dysregulated, jumping up from Dad's lap and racing across the room to find an alien figure to hold during the session. I track him verbally by saying, "Noticing hurts can be hard. Dad, Marcus feels safer if he has a toy to look at or play with while we are taking care of hurts." Marcus returns and settles back in Dad's lap. I notice a little hangnail on his hand and take care of this with some lotion. Then I notice a scar on his knee and say, "Oh, this one looks like an old hurt."

Marcus attempts to jump up again, and I shift my focus, asking a question about the weapon held by his action figure. He settles back in (the scary stuff of allowing himself to be taken care of is mitigated by his kinesthetic involvement with a toy and the shift in my focus from his physical body to his toy). I allow his neurophysiology to calm and ask his father, "Dad, it looks like this is an old hurt. Can you tell me the story of how Marcus got this hurt?" Dad is nurturing in his tone and tells the story of a time when the client ran down the driveway, going too fast, and fell and skinned his knee. Parents will often give a minimal story that supports their caretaking, such as "I got him a Band-Aid" or "I fixed him up." Our job as clinicians is to slow down the story and to help the child hear the specific caretaking actions taken by the parent. Remember, the old story for Marcus, written *in utero* and embedded over and over again in those first 2 months of detoxing in the hospital, was that there is no help for hurts.

I become curious, asking, "How did you know he was hurt?" Dad says, "Well, I heard him crying and ran onto the front porch, saw that he had fallen, and I ran down to the driveway and picked him up." I ask Dad, "What was it like to pick him up?" Dad replies, "Well, he wrapped his little arms around my neck, and I was sooo glad he trusted me to take care of him. I carried him inside, set him on the countertop, and got a paper towel with some water. I cleaned out the scrape and then I put a Band-Aid on it." I ask, "Can you show me how you did that? I have lots of Band-Aids to choose from." Dad chooses a bright blue Band-Aid and puts it over Marcus's scar. Marcus, who had been playing feverishly with his alien figure, crashing it into a tank that he had found earlier, adds, "It bleeded a lot." I say, "You remember that it bled a lot. Dad, what else did you do to help?" Dad replies, "I kissed it." I ask, "Can you show me?" Marcus is still feverishly playing with his toys and ignores the action, but Dad kisses the Band-Aid on top of Marcus's knee. I normalize the parental instinct to help boo-boos feel better, and Marcus inquires, "Can I take it off now?" I say, "Thanks for letting me know that you want that Band-Aid taken off. . . . Dad, can you take it off for him?" While the father is taking off the Band-Aid, I ask, "Dad, did Marcus run down the driveway again?" Dad says, "Yes! Once his knee had healed, he went right back to using his strong body."

This storytelling was supported in the Nurture Nook and happened near the beginning of treatment. One of the valuable lessons that Marcus's dad learned from my narration was that when his son's body begins to respond in a way that looks impulsive or dysregulated, his physiology may be communicating stress. Dad learned to say, "Your body is letting me know that . . . ," and Marcus became more secure in his ability to interpret his own body's cues and in his caregiver's ability to know what he needed. We had a series of sessions in which we engaged in rapid-fire interactions that moved from nurturing, caretaking moments to moments of intense parent–child connection that encouraged Marcus to be challenged and experience a competency surge and sense of "I can do that," followed by quiet storytelling moments. We engaged in many activities aimed at increasing his sense of connection to his parents. On one of his first visits, I introduced him to the idea of writing M's on his hand and his mom's with a Sharpie, so they could remember that they stick together even when they are apart. Marcus asked me to redraw these M's each session for many sessions after that (see Figure 9.3).

This work requires nuance and a continual focus on titration, finding the child's (and parent's) growing edge, pushing right up against the edge of their zone of proximal development, and then switching gears to fill the child's tank and reestablish optimal arousal. The therapist can sometimes feel like a ping-pong ball while doing this job. One could see it as bouncing around or as a nuanced approach to the child's scariest stuff. After several sessions like this, some with Marcus's mom and some with his dad, I requested a parent coaching session. The parents were eager to discuss some of what they were learning and to discuss their shifting paradigm. Mom showed me a photo of Marcus that had just recently been taken for school. She recognized the frozen response that was communicated through his

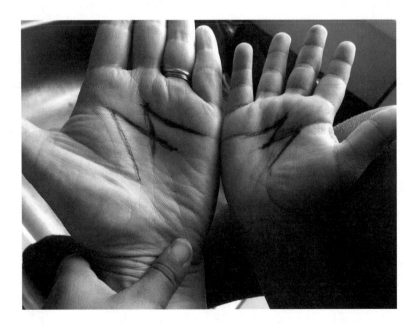

FIGURE 9.3. Connection.

blank eyes, almost grimacing smile, and rigid body. The parents expressed eagerness to help Marcus feel more comfortable in his own body and were supportive of bringing coherence to his story by tying his early withdrawal symptoms to some of his body's current ways of relating to the world.

Enhancing the Neocortext around Marcus's Birth Story

Once Marcus had deepened his healthy attachments to his parents, he was ready to hear more of his story. We used the sand tray to do this work. The sand tray serves as a powerful, boundaried space for helping families sort through the trauma, while sharing a narrative that combines words, symbols, and brings coherence and shared mindsight to family members (Carey, 1999; Homeyer & Sweeney, 2016; Malchiodi & Crenshaw, 2015; Miller & Boe, 1990). Marcus had recently asked Mom something about his birth mother, a piece of information that Mom shared in the lobby at the start of session. I am a big believer in catch-as-catch-can, and since Marcus was curious and questioning his history, I switched gears to follow his need and invited Mom to join us in the sand tray room. Trained in advanced methods for providing EMDR to children, and having used the TheraTappers previously with Marcus to further install some of his competency experiences, I went and got the buzzies. I offered to put them in his pockets or his shoes, and he chose his socks first. I asked Mom if she could pick out a figure to represent the birth mom Mandy and one to represent Marcus as a baby. We realized we needed a few other things, like a hospital bed and crib, and then Marcus blurted out (while seemingly deeply engaged with a monster truck) that we needed food, too. I made sure that a drink and a baby bottle were available, and Mom began to narrate. Mom described getting the phone call from the social worker saying that Mandy had gone into labor. Mom took the miniature that represented her, pretended to be on the phone, and said, "I'm so glad you called! I have been waiting for this moment! I'll be there as fast as I can!"

Marcus, who was playing with an action figure and listening carefully (although it may not have looked that way from an outsider's perspective), piped up and said, "Wait. The social worker?" I said, "Mom, I think it would be good to choose a figure to be the social worker, too." As Mom chose the figure, I asked her more about the social worker, and then she and I reenacted the phone call, with me assuming the voice of the social worker, calling in excitement to say that Marcus was on his way. Mandy asked that Mom stop and get a special kind of soda for her on the way to the hospital, and the client seemed reassured by this part of the story: understanding that Mom was, in her own way, taking care of his birth mom, too. Figure 9.4 shows Marcus, just born, lying on Mandy's chest. The next image (see Figure 9.5) shows the adoptive mom holding baby Marcus soon after his arrival. We all talked about how he had to stay in the hospital a long time because he was born with drugs in

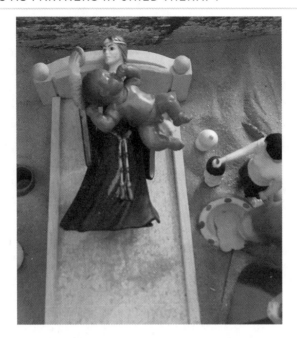

FIGURE 9.4. Birth Mom Holding Marcus.

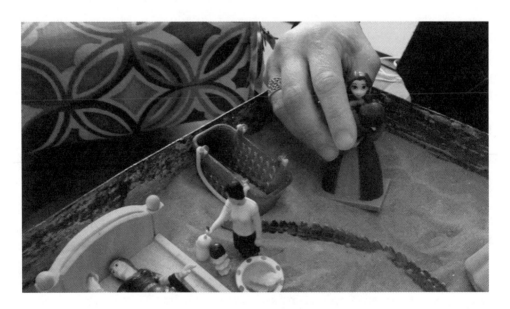

FIGURE 9.5. Adoptive Mom Holding Marcus.

his body that were making him sick. We narrated the story of his mother taking drugs and being unable to stop taking them, even while Marcus was growing in her womb. We talked about how his body had to get rid of the drugs, and it would shake and sweat and felt really sick for the first month he was alive. I wondered out loud what a little baby might start to think about how good or bad it felt to be in the world if his body wasn't able to feel better quickly. After this narration, mainly given as I asked questions of Mom and she filled in the answers, we ended by choosing other miniatures to represent the rest of his adoptive family—his dad and older siblings—who rushed to the hospital room to see him. Before he left the session, Marcus asked if we could strap the baby Marcus figure to the dad figure's chest, so I went and scrounged up a rubber band and we made sure the two figures stuck together. Marcus understood that the figures might be separated again when he returned the next week, since many children use that room, but was delighted on his return to find that the figures were still connected (see Figure 9.6). As they were leaving the room, Marcus spontaneously jumped into Mom's arms, hugging her tightly around the neck. It felt like a moment of profound connection and some gratitude for how clearly she told his story (see Figure 9.7).

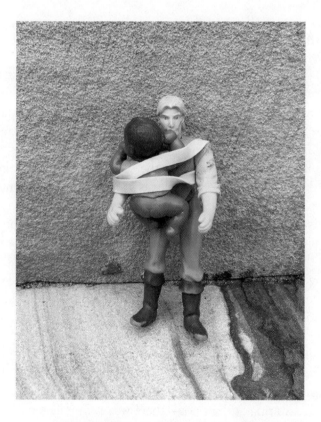

FIGURE 9.6. Dad Wearing Marcus.

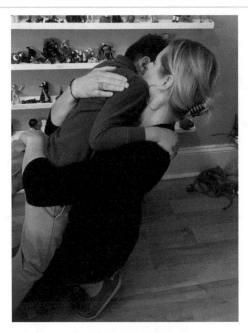

FIGURE 9.7. Spontaneous Hug after Narrative.

Working with the Activation That Arrives in the Room

It is astonishing how quickly some of our most traumatized children can shift from one set of behaviors to another, from dysregulation to regulation and back again. These fast changes of state are confusing to parents. Parents understandably believe that when they see a child rage all the way to Nurture House, screaming, yelling obscenities, and kicking the car doors, and suddenly turn it off in the lobby, this means she was in charge of her behavior the entire time and is making the choice to misbehave or to "show out" when she is alone with her parents and to then "pretend" to be "normal" and "good" when she is trying to impress others. Parents believe that this quick change translates to the child choosing to control her behavior. It may actually mean that the therapist or the new environment is more fear-inducing than the parent: The child's self-consciousness or fear of the ugliest parts of her self being seen inhibits the behaviors. Parents can benefit from a therapeutic reframe that promotes them as the safest person in the child's world . . . and therefore the one most likely to see the child in her largest, deepest moments of upset. Parents and children sometimes need help connecting the dots and making sense of the activation that arrives in the room can help.

One morning I went out to the lobby to greet Eliot and his mother. Eliot was a teenage boy adopted from Africa when he was a toddler. His mother was sitting rigidly and he was staring at the floor—there was definitely tension in the room. I escorted them into the kitchen and said, "It feels like something big just happened."

This was all the permission Mom needed to begin explaining the story: As they were walking up the path to Nurture House, Eliot asked if he could play in the playground. Mom said "yes." Eliot asked her if she would stay outside with him, and she explained that she hadn't brought a jacket and would be too cold. She immediately followed up by saying she would watch him closely through the window. Eliot melted down, screaming that she hates him and that she's a bad mom and that he should just leave this family. Mom was bewildered. As we worked with the activation, I supported Eliot in naming the feeling he was afraid of feeling in the backyard: lonely. I then asked him if he could draw the first picture that comes into his head when he feels lonely. He quietly drew the crib that you see in the far-right corner of Figure 9.8. We talked about his early time in the eerily silent baby wing of the orphanage. I asked him to draw how seeing baby Eliot in the crib made him feel, and he created a black heart on the left-hand side of the page and added the word *empty*. I then began working with the biggest parts of self for Eliot and helping big boy Eliot, along with Mom, speak to the baby and explain that he has a voice now and a mother who will listen to his words. Mom teared up while we were working, having her compassion well reopened for his deep sense of isolation. She became eager, again, to hold his story, and he gained confidence that the oldest part of himself could communicate more effectively than the baby in the crib. We went back outside and role-played their entrance onto the property, only this time when Mom indicated she would like to stay inside, Eliot said, "I think I will feel really lonely if you do that." Mom thanked him for sharing his feelings, and they came to a compromise, with her staying outside with him for a few minutes and then him coming inside to sit with her (see Figure 9.8). Tracing moments of activation within the dyad all the way back and narrating the origins of vulnerabilities in front of the parent can be helpful to both.

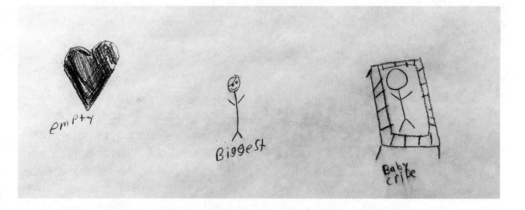

FIGURE 9.8. Youngest Self/Empty Heart.

Story-Based Psychoeducation with Parents

Tanika, a 3-year-old girl, was adopted from an orphanage in a third world country 2 years ago. Her adoptive parents also have a biological child who is 2 years old. They requested a session because they were seeing massive differences between the two children. Tanika was born and left under a bridge. She was found and taken to the orphanage. At 12 months old, Tanika was sleeping in a room with many other children. She slept on a thin mattress on the floor so that if she fell off, she would just roll onto the floor. Tanika would get up in the middle of the night and move from bed to bed, holding out her hand for high fives. Once she found someone who was awake enough to high five her back, she would crawl up into bed with that person. In that way, she worked very hard to get this basic need for touch and physical comfort met using the resources that were available to her. Ten minutes prior to the end of the session, after several key concepts related to trauma (the amygdala alarm, bottom-up brain development) had been explored, Dad described his daughter's tendency to wake up revved. He said, "She's got the kind of alarm clock that turns green at 6:30 A.M. I'm never sure how long she has been up, but she is always standing and staring at the clock for the moment that it turns green and then she is out of there. Is that a trauma thing?" Dad and I put on our curiosity caps and wondered together about the underlying need being expressed. Pulling the threads of Tanika's early life through her development, to the present moment, opened up our compassion wells. We agreed that Tanika was saying, "I need to be near you."

Bring It in the Room

Helping parents change cycles of communication with their children and with each other requires that first we really work to understand the cycle. Understanding the cycle requires calling attention to it, with curiosity and compassion, when we see problematic or confusing communication happening. In TraumaPlay supervision, we talk about this process as Bringing *It* in the Room. Which begs the question, what is the "it"?

The "It"

The *It* can take many forms, but represents the identified moment in which one person's communication triggers another's. The *It* can be interpersonal or intrapersonal. Interpersonally, the *It* may show up as a subtle, nonverbal tightening of the jaw for a parent when a child begins to whine in session. The *It* may show up as a parent smiling at a moment that seems incongruent with the content being explored with the child in play, sand, art, or words at the time. Intrapersonally, a parent may become blank or seem to have "checked out" during an interaction. Noticing this response and asking the parent what was going on inside at that time can lead to rich reflection with the parent on his own Window of Tolerance for engaged play, for confrontation, for remaining present, and so on. Sometimes the *It* is a parent's acceptance of a child's miscue. Trauma-informed caregiving requires the parent to understand the miscue as the way the child has chosen to cope with earlier unmet needs or overwhelming emotions instead of taking the communication at face value. One of the most devastating parent–child interaction cycles is that in which the attachment-disrupted child miscues the parent that she doesn't need any help, that she can do and prefers to do everything for herself. The parent who takes these cues at face value may miss rich opportunities to help that child push through the risk of trusting someone to help her.

Intrapersonal processes can also be explored with the child or teen during a parent–child session. A seasoned clinician in our group TraumaPlay supervision recently shared a powerful example that highlights the need to focus on bringing intrapersonal process into the room. In TraumaPlay, we are often working on parallel tracks to help traumatized children learn to soothe their own physiology, utilizing various playful biofeedback tools, while simultaneously training parents to co-regulate their children's physiology more effectively. This clinician had been working with a family for some time and had established a strong therapeutic alliance with both Mom and the client. She had also taught Joey (age 6, internationally adopted) how to use the stethoscope, the oximeter, and the heart rate app on her phone to see how fast his heart was beating at various points in treatment. Previously, this biofeedback work was only used when the treatment goal was focused on expanding the young man's Window of Tolerance for various states of arousal. He would engage in an upregulating activity, take his pulse, and then engage in a play-based form of downregulation and take his pulse again. He was gratified to learn that he had more influence over his internal state of being than he had previously understood.

In this particular session, Mom, client, and therapist had all been dancing together, increasing their heart rates and comparing notes on how fast their hearts were beating. The therapist then invited Joey and Mom to snuggle together, while Mom read a book to him. Mom picked the classic children's book *The Runaway Bunny* from the shelf and began reading it. For those readers who may not be familiar with the narrative's format, one page sets up an attempt by the bunny to run away from the momma bunny. One page says, "I will become a crocus in a hidden garden," and then the momma bunny responds, "If you became a crocus in a hidden garden, I would become a gardener and I would water you." Over and over again, the baby bunny concocts scenarios in which he would be separated from Mom and Mom becomes whatever she needs to in order to remain close to her baby. Because the oximeter was still on Joey's finger, we were able to notice a pattern that we had not understood before: While the posture of Joey's body remained relaxed, even molded against mom's, and his facial expression remained neutral throughout the reading, his heart rate increased significantly on the pages where the bunny ran away, and would slow when Mom read the mommy bunny's strategy for making sure she could stay with him. This session was remarkable and afforded an opportunity, due to the external monitoring of internal states, to see his body's interoception of safety, during what his body perceived as the threat of the little bunny's separation from Mom. The clinician, grounded in the Bring It in the Room mantra, said, "Your body was telling us some really important things while we were reading that book! When the baby bunny talked about running away, your heart rate went up . . . that's the body's way of letting us know that something is exciting or scary. I wouldn't have known by looking at you that your heart was beating faster—your face and body still looked so relaxed. Mom, I'm wondering if this happens other times, too. Joey's inside body is telling him that he's stressed in some way, but his outside is saying that he's fine. I bet this has helped Joey in the past, but now that he's with you, I think it would be really helpful for us all to learn more about what Joey's body is telling him and how so that we can help more quickly whenever he needs it."

This clinician had already begun to develop a trauma-informed hypothesis that Joey had learned early on, in his institutional environment, to pretend that he was calm and confident even when he was really scared. Neither the staff nor the other children had patience for crying, screaming, or distressed children, so he had just learned to mask his distress. However, the body does indeed "keep the score" (van der Kolk, 2015), and in this case, the continual incongruence between Joey's internal upset and external calm was keeping him from being soothed by his adoptive mother and from helping him learn to soothe himself. Trauma therapists learn to titrate their approach to the scary thing (Goodyear-Brown, 2019). In this case, the core fear and need that Joey had learned to mask would need to eventually become shared narrative, but some work on internal congruence could begin in a very playful way right away. The clinician talked with Joey and his mom about becoming detectives together and learning to understand what Joey's body was telling him about excitement and fear. In supervision, we discussed playful, low-stress ways to curiously "watch" how his body responded to new stimuli. We created a menu of tactile experiences, including putting his hands in a bowl of spaghetti, rubbing his hands along soft flannel, and experiencing a hug from Mom (all with the oximeter on), so that we could record his heart rate during each of these experiences. Eventually, Joey will be able to predict how his heart rate will respond to various kinds of new situations and further predict what he needs to decrease his heart rate. The wake of Joey's competency surges brought about by accurately attuning to his internal states mitigates the approach to the more difficult content. We can enlist Mom to help hold the hard parts of his story.

As an attachment therapist, I love the richness of metaphor in *The Runaway Baby*. The momma bunny and her son give voice to the overarching complexity of every child's need for separation in order to grow identity, independence, and sense of self and every mother's need for adaptability and flexibility in accepting their fantastical self-definition and burgeoning autonomy. The little boy bunny is asking throughout, *Can I become? How will it affect us if I become?* The momma bunny's unspoken question, *How do I maintain connection during his individuation?*, is solved by simply becoming whatever is needed to continue to nurture and guide him. In each iteration, she is staying close enough, in terms of physical proximity, to provide safety while still allowing him to try out different roles. Although this book can be seen as charming, or even tender and hopeful to a dyad in which the mother has met the baby's every need since infancy, it is a terrifying scenario for Joey. He missed those thousands and thousands of repetitions of need meeting that happen in the first 3 years of life, not arriving home until he was three-and-a-half. At just about the age when he would be hitting rapprochement and individuating, he is instead faced with the much earlier developmental task of attaching. All of those interactions that begin developing a child's sense of object permanency (the understanding that something exists even when you can't see it) were denied to him. Crafting a story around this early experience that includes Mom's role now will be important for Joey.

Needed Narration

Johnny was a young man who looked like he was 14 although he was only 9 years old. This made his core developmental struggle even more difficult. Johnny was also a young man who had been adopted domestically soon after birth, but he had been sick *in utero* and was born very ill. When he was referred, he was raging uncontrollably at home, and his parents were unsure how to continue moving forward with him. Johnny needed to have his story recapitulated with his adoptive mother in order to move forward. Some of this client's story is published in *Go With That Magazine,* a publication of the EMDR International Association (EMDRIA). When Johnny came in one day enacting patterns that were clearly echoes of his early neglect, I decided it was important that we narrate some of his early life. I asked Mom if she could create a sand tray that showed me her earliest memory of him. Mom gathered her figures, while Johnny hid most of his body on one side of a giant exercise ball: Only his eyes could be seen above it, carefully watching the construction of the sand tray.

As we spoke about Johnny's birth, Mom explained that when she arrived to pick him up, he was lying on a hospital bed, only wearing a diaper; she instantly wondered if he was cold in just his diaper. I wondered out loud what kind of blanket would have been a good covering and offered several small swatches of cloth. Johnny pointed to one and became, in that moment, invested in taking care of the baby in the story—the self-object that needed nurturing. Children who come from hard places often need to absorb nurture vicariously at first by observing the way in which the therapist takes care of the chosen self-object, before they are able to receive nurture directly from the therapist (Goodyear-Brown, 2010). After Johnny pointed to the cloth, I offered it to Mom, who tucked it in, ever so carefully, around the baby in the hospital bed. I then said, "Show me what it was like to take him home from the hospital." Johnny began to roll the top half of his body onto the exercise ball, rolling closer to the sand tray and then away again. I said, "We need to pack a bag for home, Mom!" I usually address a client's parents as "Mom" and "Dad" instead of using their first names while narrating things related to their care-giving, especially for children who are not yet convinced that their mother or father actually functions in the role of mother or father. Mom said, "Yes, he will need a blanket, a bottle. . . ." Johnny joined in at this point and said, "and a pacifier!" I smiled at Johnny and made sure that we had a pacifier "packed" for the baby's trip home. Since then, we have been able to tell more stories of Johnny's most recent, big boy adventures. We have often done this while he regulates on the swing. Most recently, after a day of successful growth of his courage on the swing, he painted a picture of the tree, the grass, and the swing (see Figure 9.9). The smiling face is his. When I asked him about the google eyes, he said, "That is you guys watching me." Once he was experiencing strong mastery play on the swing, we began titrating doses of approach to harder content.

We have narrated, at Nurture House, many a home-going. We have reenacted parents getting on a plane with rubles to go get their child from Russia, as the child watches intently from behind the sand tray. We have narrated the moment at which an Asian woman watched for hours for the right couple to take her child—and then placed her daughter directly in their path as they walked along the river bank, to ensure that the baby be raised by people whom she had chosen to love her.

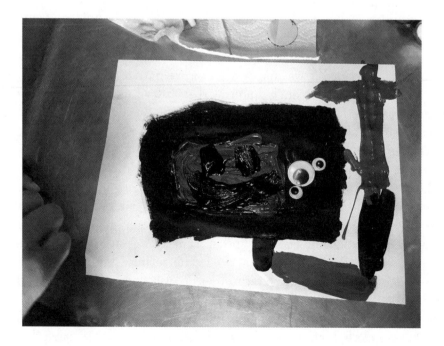

FIGURE 9.9. Seeing Me.

Encouraging Emotional Integration

For Alicia, who has always had difficulty naming the feelings that are harder for her, this difficulty was amplified when her parents worked their way toward divorce. Now that her parents have officially filed for divorce, she is experiencing an almost full-time nanny in one home, while that parent works inordinately long shifts to try to ensure that the same financial resources as before will remain available to the children, while also moving to a rhythm of life in which she only sees the other parent much less frequently.

All of the tension mounting between her parents culminated one afternoon during a music lesson. Mom had brought Alicia to a music lesson, during her parenting time, and afterward Dad had called—repeatedly—while they were waiting for a sibling to finish a lesson. With many children also in the waiting room, Dad showed up and began yelling and saying negative things to Mom. The children watched as the very uncomfortable interaction unfolded. Remember that in TraumaPlay, we believe very strongly in letting children know what we know about the hard thing that has happened, so during Alicia's next session, I brought her into the sand tray room and said, "Mom called to let me know that there was a hard moment after your piano lesson, where Dad came in and yelled at Mom in the lobby." Instead of asking her a question about how she felt, I simply said, "I imagine you had lots of big feelings about what happened." I said this while smoothing out the sand in the tray with my open palm. Alicia was watching my hand moving back and forth in the tray when she offered, "I guess I'm just used to it. I don't really care." Then I asked a question: "So what do you feel when you think about what happened?" Alicia said, "Nothing, really." I offered Alicia the Mixed-Emotion Cards and she rolled her eyes. I said, "Flip through all the cards and choose three that catch your eye when you think about being at the piano lesson, sitting on the bench, listening to one of your parents yelling at the other while the people sitting nearby watch."

Alicia and I had been working together for a year at this point, so although she liked to express her displeasure with eye rolling, she trusted me deeply and was willing to engage. I made the activity a little more fun by telling her that she could hide the cards in the room as she chose each one and then I would have to find them. She spent a great deal of time sorting through the cards and finally chose three. We developed a game in which she would give different eye signals for "hot" and "cold" as I moved around the room, helping me to find her hidden feelings. The feelings she identified were *stressed, confused,* and *unsure.* I had her set each of the three cards upright in the sand tray . . . and then we just absorbed them for a few minutes. Eventually, I said, "Do you think you could pick a symbol to represent each of the three feeling cards you displayed here?" She grinned and said, "I'm way ahead of you" which was probably true given that she had been my client for awhile and knew my propensity for fleshing out left-brain linguistic narrative with right-brain, Gestalt-ish symbolism. She chose a figure that had ironically been created by another child, a clay head with tufts of fiery hair attached—the figure looked almost like a brain on fire—and settled it in the sand in front of the card that said "stressed." Alicia searched for a long time for the second symbol, but chose a tornado to represent the sense of "confusion" she felt about her parent's divorce and the resulting animosity between them. Part of her confusion centered around the two different explanations she had been given about why the yelling happened. The two versions did not line up, and Alicia was left feeling unsure about whom she should believe. The final card that Alicia had chosen, which read "unsure," depicts two different streets at a crossroads. Alicia looked intently at the shelves for a long period of time and then chose the three triplets from *Brave*: the three red-headed boys who were always fairly rambunctious. Fascinating—not one self, not two selves, but three. Internally, I wondered if she has two different kinds of self that she shows, one to Mom and one to Dad, and I hoped that the third self represented a true self that Alicia was on a journey to defining.

Garden Timelines

Often children and teens present to counseling burdened by an overwhelming history of stressful and negative life events. The pressures of such events can eradicate memories of strengths and personal victories, causing them instead to adapt an incoherent and cynical narrative of their life story. Play therapy and the narrative approach blend beautifully to help bring incongruent parts of a child's story together through artistic and expressive mediums. Children can find relief from the burden of a traumatic narrative by witnessing their story, integrating the trauma, and making sense of these life experiences in the context of a safe and supportive therapeutic environment.

One play-based way of helping a child witness her story and develop a coherent narrative is through the creation of a Garden Timeline. This visual representation of a child's life story serves not only as a visual container for the entirety of her story, but also as a titration medium for exposure to deeper work.

This intervention begins by providing a developmentally appropriate rationale for narrative and story work, highlighting the importance and value of one's unique story and the ways in which life events can shape who we are. The metaphor of a garden can be applied to a life story by highlighting the fact that both require a process and gradually unfold with the passing of time. Just as seeds are planted, sometimes life events are planted into our lives, and the type of garden that is created is reflective of the seeds it holds. I will often mention that maintaining a garden, clearing weeds, and nurturing its growth through proper amounts of sun and rain are hard but important work, just like taking care of ourselves through the counseling process. Frequently, maintaining the integrity of a garden requires that we look deeper and notice any barriers impeding its growth, such as rocks, stones, or unhealthy soil. I will always validate that everyone has stones or places of unhealthy soil in their "garden" story. Some have more or less than others, but everyone has the responsibility of taking care of their own garden. Once the metaphor has been established, the child is invited to begin creating her own Garden Timeline. A long piece of butcher paper is cut and a line or long piece of colored tape is placed down the middle of the paper, dividing it into an upper and lower half. At the far end of the line, the therapist writes the child's birthday, signifying the beginning of her life story. From there, the child describes the events in her life, good and bad, in chronological order. For every good memory, the child creates a flower stem with a flower and glues it above the line. This could be a positive experience, life addition, or meaningful person in her life. The child chooses to create a short or tall stem based on how "positive" that memory feels to her. The therapist describes the positive life event on the stem of the flower, and the child creates a flower top of her choice. For every bad memory, such as a death, loss, person, or traumatic event, the child glues a paper stone cut out beneath the line and can choose the size of the stone based on how negative or "heavy" that memory feels to her. The therapist labels the stone based on the identification provided by the child. For the memories that feel particularly "stuck" or "unclear" for the child, she is invited to glue a mud puddle below the line, reflecting a stuck part in her story, which the therapist also labels. Once the child has recounted her life story and created her chronological

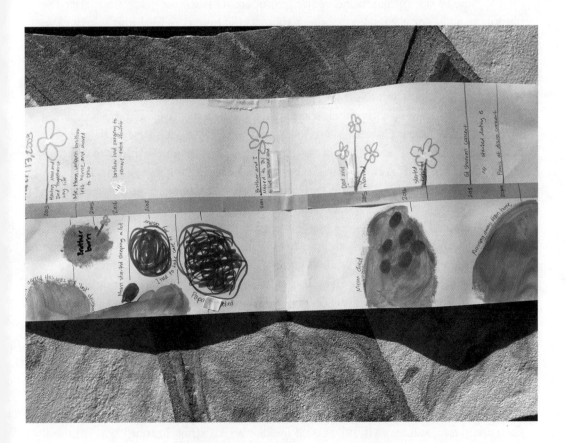

FIGURE 9.10. Example Garden Timeline.

Garden Timeline, the child and therapist reflect on it together, noticing themes, resilience, and seasons of significance throughout the client's life story.

Through this creative engagement with a child's life narrative, the child is able to recount her significant life events in a safe setting, reexperience emotions connected to those events, and engage with them in a new way. Not only does this process help a child learn that she can engage with memories and not become dysregulated by them, but she also learns the redemptive beauty of a story with many different parts that comes together with purpose and meaning. Children are empowered to notice the beauty in their stories when everything can seem like dirt. An example of a Garden Timeline is given in Figure 9.10.

I'm Still Standing

There are certain clients that you walk with for years. This is the story of one of mine. Thomas was a toddler when I met him. His paternal grandfather had sought me out and arranged for an initial session that included all four grandparents. Thomas's parents were both engaged in addictive behaviors and were in and out of his life. At the time of the intake, none of the grandparents held out much hope that the parents would ever get back custody of their son. Thomas held things pretty close to the vest and would quietly build sand trays full of dinosaurs. Often the dinosaurs would develop factions, they would fight, there would be casualties, and then the whole war would start again. I had intermittent contact with Thomas's mother, who loved him very much, but felt trapped within controlling and dysfunctional patterns in her family of origin, with which she coped by self-medicating. Thomas's dad had not been given a clear place in his son's life and was making self-destructive choices of his own. At some point in the cycles of addiction, rehab, and wanting to connect more deeply with his son, Thomas's dad started coming for parent coaching sessions. I worked hard to show him the kind of father he could be, and several times over the course of those years, as bitter disappointments occurred, he would drop out, or be forced out, of his son's life. Through a series of events that involved sudden trauma and the growth that can often result from suffering, both parents began making different choices and worked hard to consistently parent Thomas, prove to the court that they were drug-free, and begin to take daily care of Thomas. They honored, to the letter of the court orders, the stipulations that someone else be present in the home overnight until the court believed they had proved themselves to be safe and consistent caregivers. In the culmination of 3 years of walking with this little boy through separations and reunions with either or both of his parents, the courts granted Mom and Dad joint custody.

In the first session following the court's decision, Thomas upon arrival confidently said, "I need markers and paper." He drew and he drew, five pages in all, and then asked for a stapler so that he could make a book. When his book was finished, he asked to go outside and said, "Now I'm gonna be the teacher and you be the class." He sat in the swinging chair and began his story. "First there was a desert and there was a helicopter, but it had no place to land. [He gestured to the image in Figure 9.11.] After a long time, there was a peaceful land [see Figure 9.12]."

Thomas went on to weave in a couple of images from *Spider-Man: Far From Home,* since he had recently seen this film, the last of which was a picture of Lava Man. He had also done a kinetic family drawing that he added as the last page of his book. He said, "Lava Man came after them, but the family jumped in the RTV and rode away" (see Figure 9.13). Once Thomas was done reading the story, he jumped down and said, "I wanna go swing!" We moved over to the magic carpet swing, and he lay down on his stomach. The swing is pictured in Figure 9.14.

He asked to be pushed while lying down on his stomach. I reflected that it sort of looked as if he was flying. Thomas grinned and scooched himself toward the front of the swing facing me and put his fists out like Superman. After awhile he said, "That's high enough. I'm gonna try it different." I encouraged him to tightly hold onto the cords, and he struggled up to his knees. It seemed to feel scary to him; we then had the following exchange:

PARIS: You did it! Looks like it felt a little scary, but you did it!

THOMAS: (*with a big grin on his face*) Yep. I'm gonna try standing up. . . .

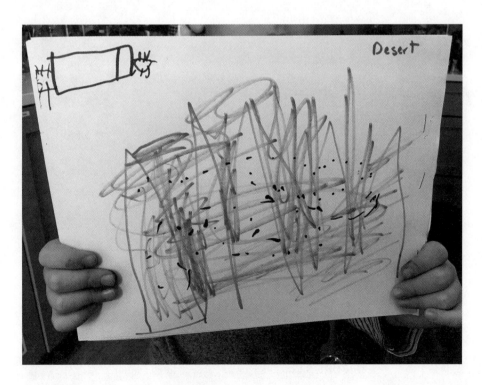

FIGURE 9.11. A Desert Land.

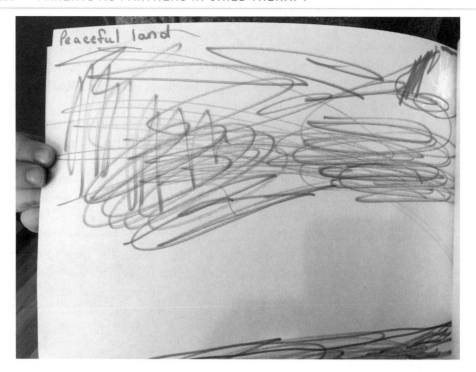

FIGURE 9.12. A Peaceful Land.

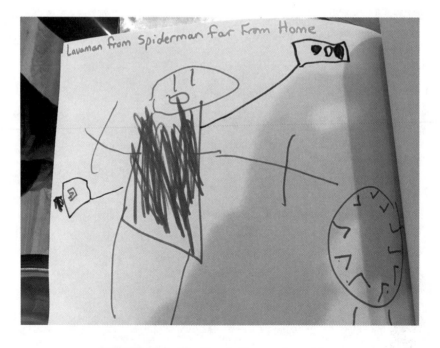

FIGURE 9.13. The Family Escapes Lava Man.

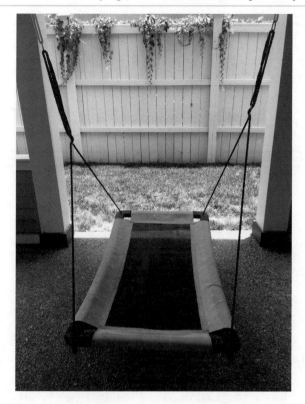

FIGURE 9.14. Magic Carpet Swing.

I watched him as he seemed to visibly gather his courage, and he wobbled his way up into a standing position. When he had struggled to a standing position, I said, "You did it!"

THOMAS: This reminds me of that song, "I'm Still Standing"!

PARIS: (*feeling the impact of the lyrics already on Thomas's situation*) I know that song. It's Elton John. I'm gonna find it and play it while you swing.

I found the version of this song from the children's movie *Sing* and played it. It's hard to describe the intensity of emotion communicated and the celebratory exhale we took together as he swung with abandon and we sang the lyrics at the top of our lungs together. Whenever we got to the chorus and got to repeat the phrase "I'm still standing," he would swing higher. When I shared this story with Mom and Dad, we all teared up together, grateful that after 3 years of these parents working hard to become a family, they had become Safe Bosses, Nurturers, and Storykeepers for this precious boy.

I wanted to leave you with this story of peace and reunification occurring after so much pain had been experienced by everyone in the system. You have the great

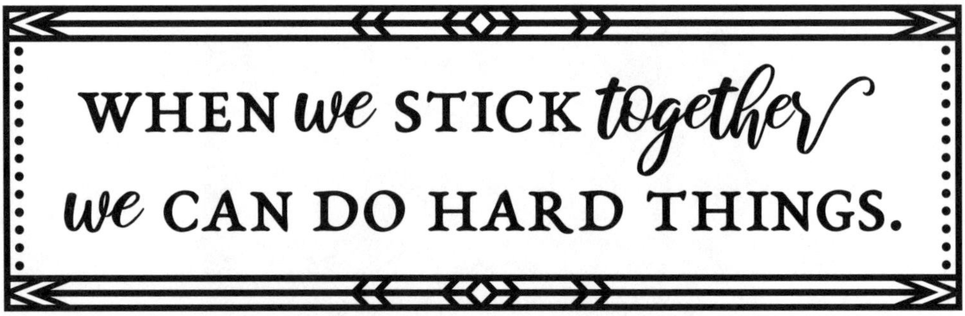

FIGURE 9.15. When We Stick Together Mantra.

privilege of being a Storykeeper for the families in your care, even as you are growing the parents' storykeeping capacity. I'd like to end this text in the way I began it—with great hope that when we stick together, helping parents and children to do the same, we can do hard things. We can do the hardest thing while continuing to grow together. I have included one final handout (see Figure 9.15). Feel free to offer it to the families in your care as they are graduating. It is a simple reminder of the truth: "When we stick together, we can do hard things." That goes for child therapists and parent coaches, too!

References

Ainsworth, M. D. S., & Bell, S. M. (1970). Attachment, exploration, and separation: Illustrated by the behavior of one-year-olds in a strange situation. *Child Development, 41*(1), 49–67.

Anda, R. F., Felitti, V. J., Bremner, J. D., Walker, J. D., Whitfield, C., Perry, B. D., et al. (2006). The enduring effects of abuse and related adverse experiences in childhood: A convergence of evidence from neurobiology and epidemiology. *European Archives of Psychiatry and Clinical Neuroscience, 256*(3), 174–186.

Applegate, J. S., & Shapiro, J. R. (2005). *Neurobiology for clinical social work: Theory and practice.* New York: Norton.

Badenoch, B. (2008). *Being a brain-wise therapist: A practical guide to interpersonal neurobiology.* New York: Norton.

Badenoch, B., & Kestly, T. (2015). Exploring the neuroscience of healing play at every age. In D. Crenshaw & A. Stewart (Eds.), *Play therapy: A comprehensive guide to theory and practice* (pp. 524–538). New York: Guilford Press.

Bailey, R. A. (2015). *Conscious discipline: Building resilient classrooms.* Loving Guidance.

Baumrind, D. (1989). Rearing competent children. In W. Damon (Ed.), *Child development today and tomorrow* (pp. 349–378). San Francisco: Jossey-Bass.

Berk, L. S., Felten, D. L., Tan, S. A., Bittman, B. B., & Westengard, J. (2001). Modulation of neuroimmune parameters during the eustress of humor-associated mirthful laughter. *Alternative Therapies in Health and Medicine, 7*(2), 62–76.

Booth, P. B., & Jernberg, A. M. (2010). *Theraplay: Helping parents and children build better relationships through attachment-based play* (3rd ed.). San Francisco: Jossey-Bass.

Bowlby, J. (1969). *Attachment and loss: Vol.1. Attachment.* New York: Basic Books.

Bowlby, J. (1973). *Separation: Anxiety and anger: Vol. 2. Attachment and loss.* London: Hogarth Press.

Bowlby, J. (1980). *Loss: Sadness and depression: Vol. 3. Attachment and loss.* London: Hogarth Press.

Bowlby, J. (1988). *A secure base: Parent–child attachment and healthy human development.* London: Routledge.

Brown, B. (2015). *Daring greatly.* New York: Avery Press.

Burke, C. A. (2010). Mindfulness-based approaches with children and adolescents: A preliminary review of current research in an emergent field. *Journal of Child and Family Studies, 19*(2), 133–144.

Carey, L. (1999). *Sandplay therapy with children and families.* Lanham, MD: Rowman & Littlefield.

Chapman, G. (1995). *The five languages of love.* Chicago: Northfield.

Cicchetti, D., Rogosch, F. A., & Toth, S. L. (2006). Fostering secure attachment in infants in maltreating families through preventive interventions. *Development and Psychopathology, 18,* 623–649.

Colandro, L. (2014). *There was an old lady who swallowed a fly!* New York: Scholastic.

Courtney, A. J. (2014). Overview of touch related to professional ethical and clinical practice with children. In J. A. Courtney & N. D. Nolan (Eds.), *Touch in child counseling and play therapy: An ethical guide* (pp. 3–18). New York: Routledge.

Dewdney, A. (2015). *Llama llama red pajama.* New York: Viking.

Dunbar, R. I. (2010). The social role of touch in humans and primates: Behavioural function and neurobiological mechanisms. *Neuroscience and Biobehavioral Reviews, 34,* 260–268.

Dunn, W. (2007). Supporting children to participate successfully in everyday life by using sensory processing knowledge. *Infants and Young Children, 20*(2), 84–101.

Erikson, E. H. (1993). *Childhood and society.* New York: Norton.

Faber, A., & Mazlish, E. (1980/2012). *How to talk so kids will listen and listen so kids will talk.* New York: Scribner.

Feldman, R., & Eidelman, A. I. (2007). Maternal postpartum behavior and the emergence of infant–mother and infant–father synchrony in preterm and full-term infants: The role of neonatal vagal tone. *Developmental Psychobiology, 49,* 290–302.

Field, T. (2019). Social touch, CT touch and massage therapy: A narrative review. *Developmental Review, 51,* 123–145.

Field, T., Diego, M., & Hernandez-Reif, M. (2007). Massage therapy research. *Developmental Review, 27,* 75–89.

Field, T., Schanberg, S. M., Scafidi, F., Bauer, C. R., Vega Lahr, N., Garcia, R., et al. (1986). Tactile/kinesthetic stimulation effects on preterm neonates. *Pediatrics, 77,* 654–658.

Fonagy, P., Gergely, G., Jurist, E., & Target, M. (2002). *Affect regulation, mentalization, and the development of the self.* New York: Brunner-Routledge.

Fosha, D. (2003). Dyadic regulation and experiential work with emotions and relatedness in trauma and disorganized attachment. In M. F. Solomon & D. J. Siegel (Eds.), *Healing trauma: Attachment, mind, body, and brain* (pp. 221–281). New York: Norton.

Fox, E. (2016). The use of humor in family therapy: Rationale and applications. *Journal of Family Psychotherapy, 27*(1), 67–78.

Franzini, L. R. (2001). Humor in therapy: The case for training therapists in its uses and risks. *Journal of General Psychology, 128*(2), 170–193.

Fries, A. B., & Pollak, S. D. (2004). Emotion understanding in postinstitutionalized Eastern European children. *Development and Psychopathology, 16*(2), 355–369.

Fritz, H. L., Russek, L. N., & Dillon, M. M. (2017). Humor use moderates the relation of stressful life events with psychological distress. *Personality and Social Psychology Bulletin, 43*(6), 845–859.

Fry, W. F., Jr., & Salameh, W. A. (Eds.). (1987). *Handbook of humor and psychotherapy: Advances in the clinical use of humor.* Sarasota, FL: Professional Resource Exchange.

Garrick, J. (2005). The humor of trauma survivors: Its application in a therapeutic milieu. *Journal of Aggression, Maltreatment and Trauma, 12*(1), 169–182.

Garrick, J. (2014). The humor of trauma survivors: Its application in a therapeutic milieu. In J. Garrick & M. C. Williams (Eds.), *Trauma treatment techniques* (pp. 169–182). New York: Routledge.

Gaskill, R., & Perry, B. (2012). Child abuse, traumatic experiences, and their impact on the developing brain. In P. Goodyear-Brown (Ed.), *Handbook of child sexual abuse* (pp. 29–67). Hoboken, NJ: Wiley.

Gaskill, R. L., & Perry, B. (2014). The neurobiological power of play: Using the neurosequential model of therapeutics to guide play in the healing process. In C. A. Malchiodi & D. A. Crenshaw (Eds.), *Creative arts and play therapy for attachment problems* (pp. 178–194). New York: Guilford Press.

George, C., Kaplan, N., & Main, M. (1985). *Adult Attachment Interview.* Unpublished manuscript, Department of Psychology, University of California, Berkeley. Retrieved from *www.psychology.sunysb.edu/attachment/measures/content/aai_interview.pdf.*

George, C., Kaplan, N., & Main, M. (1996). *Adult Attachment Interview* (3rd ed.). Unpublished manuscript, Department of Psychology, University of California, Berkeley. Retrieved from *http://library.allanschore.com/docs/AAIProtocol.pdf.*

Gil, E. (2014). *Play in family therapy.* New York: Guilford Press.

Gladding, S. T., & Drake Wallace, M. J. (2016). Promoting beneficial humor in counseling: A way of helping counselors help clients. *Journal of Creativity in Mental Health, 11*(1), 2–11.

Glynn, L. M., & Sandman, C. A. (2011). Prenatal origins of neurological development: A critical period for fetus and mother. *Current Directions in Psychological Science, 20*(6), 384–389.

Goldin, E., Bordan, T., Araoz, D. L., Gladding, S. T., Kaplan, D., Krumboltz, J., et al. (2006). Humor in counseling: Leader perspectives. *Journal of Counseling and Development, 84*(4), 397–404.

Goleman, D. (2006). *Emotional intelligence: Why it can matter more than IQ.* New York: Bantam.

Gomez, A. (2012). *EMDR therapy and adjunct approaches to complex trauma, attachment, and dissociation.* New York: Springer.

Goodyear-Brown, P. (2002). *Digging for buried treasure: 52 prop-based play therapy interventions for treating the problems of childhood.* Nashville, TN: Author.

Goodyear-Brown, P. (2010a). *Play therapy with traumatized children.* Hoboken, NJ: Wiley.

Goodyear-Brown, P. (2010b). The worry wars. Retrieved from *www.parisgoodyearbrown.com.*

Goodyear-Brown, P. (2011). The worry wars: A protocol for treating childhood anxiety disorders. In A. A. Drewes, S. C. Bratton, & C. E. Schaefer (Eds.), *Integrative play therapy* (pp. 129–152). Hoboken, NJ: Wiley.

Goodyear-Brown, P. (2013). Tackling touchy subjects. Retrieved from *www.parisgoodyearbrown.com.*

Goodyear-Brown, P. (2019a). *Trauma and play therapy: Helping children heal.* New York: Routledge.

Goodyear-Brown, P. (2019b, March). Parents as partners: Enhancing co-regulation and coherence though an integration of play therapy and EMDR. *Go With That EMDRIA Magazine*, 28–33. Retrieved from *https://issuu.com/emdriagwt/docs/emdria_march_2019_magazine__3_*.

Goodyear-Brown, P. (2020). Prescriptive play therapy for attachment disruptions in children. In H. G. Kaduson, D. Cangelosi, & C. E. Schaefer (Eds.), *Prescriptive play therapy: Tailoring interventions for specific childhood* (pp. 231–250). New York: Guilford Press.

Goodyear-Brown, P., & Andersen, E. (2018). Play therapy for separation anxiety in children. In A. A. Drewes & C. Schaefer (Eds.), *Play-based interventions for childhood anxieties, fears, and phobias* (pp. 158–176). New York: Guilford Press.

Graves-Alcorn, S. L., & Green, E. (2014). The expressive arts therapy continuum: History and theory. In E. Green & A. A. Drewes (Eds.), *Integrating expressive arts and play therapy with children and adolescents* (pp. 1–16). Hoboken, NJ: Wiley.

Graves-Alcorn, S. L., & Kagin, C. (2017). *Implementing the expressive therapies continuum: A guide for clinical practice*. New York: Routledge.

Hasan, H., & Hasan, T. F. (2009). Laugh yourself into a healthier person: A cross-cultural analysis of the effects of varying levels of laughter on health. *International Journal of Medical Sciences, 6*(4), 200–211.

Hatigan, J. D., Lambert, B. L., Seifer, R., Ekas, N. V., Bauer, C. R., & Messinger, D. S. (2012). Security of attachment and quality of mother–toddler social interaction in a high-risk sample. *Infant Behavior and Development, 35*, 83–93.

Hebb, D. (1949). *The organization of behavior*. New York: Wiley.

Hembree-Kigin, T. L., & McNeil, C. B. (2013). *Parent–child interaction therapy*. New York: Springer.

Hoffman, K., Cooper, G., Powell, B., & Benton, C. (2017). *Raising a secure child: How Circle of Security parenting can help you nurture your child's attachment, emotional resilience, and freedom to explore*. New York: Guilford Press.

Homeyer, L. E., & Sweeney, D. S. (2016). *Sand tray therapy: A practical manual* (2nd ed.). New York: Routledge.

Hong, R., & Mason, C. M. (2016). Becoming a neurobiologically-informed play therapist. *International Journal of Play Therapy, 25*(1), 35–44.

Hughes, D., & Baylin, J. (2012). *Brain-based parenting: The neuroscience of caregiving for healthy attachment*. New York: Norton.

Isen, A. M. (2003). Positive affect as a source of human strength. In L. G. Aspinwall & U. M. Staudinger (Eds.), *A psychology of human strengths: Fundamental questions and future directions for positive psychology* (pp. 179–195). Washington, DC: American Psychological Association.

Jackson, J. H. (1958). Evolution and dissolution of the nervous system. In J. J. Taylor (Ed.), *Selected writings of John Hughlings Jackson* (pp. 45–118). London: Staples Press.

Jung, C. G. (1939). *The integration of the personality*. New York: Farrar & Rinehart.

Kabat-Zinn, J. (2003). Mindfulness-based interventions in context: Past, present, and future. *Clinical Psychology: Science and Practice, 10*, 144–156.

Kay, J. (2009). Toward a neurobiology of child psychotherapy. *Journal of Loss and Trauma, 14*, 287–303.

Kestly, T. (2015). *The interpersonal neurobiology of play: Brain-building interventions for emotional well-being.* New York: Norton.

Kirsch, P., Esslinger, C., Chen, Q., Mier, D., Lis, S., Siddhanti, S., et al. (2005). Oxytocin modulates neural circuitry for social cognition and fear in humans. *Journal of Neuroscience, 25*(49), 11489–11493.

Kranowitz, S. C. (2005). *The out-of-sync child: Recognizing and coping with sensory processing disorder.* New York: Berkley.

Landgarten, H. B. (1987). *Family art psychotherapy: A clinical guide and casebook.* New York: Brunner/Mazel.

Landreth, G. (2002). *Play therapy: The art of the relationship* (2nd ed.). New York: Brunner-Routledge.

LeDoux, J. E. (1996). *The emotional brain.* New York: Simon & Schuster.

Lowenfeld, M. (1950) The nature and use of the Lowenfeld world technique in work with children and adults. *Journal of Psychology, 30,* 325–331.

MacLean, P. D. (1990). *The triune brain in evolution: Role of paleocerebral functions.* New York: Plenum Press.

Main, M., & Cassidy, J. (1988). Categories of response to reunion with the parent at age 6: Predictable from infant attachment classifications and stable over a 1-month period. *Developmental Psychology, 24*(3), 415.

Main, M., Hesse, E., & Kaplan, N. (2005). Predictability of attachment behavior and representational processes at 1, 6, and 18 years of age: The Berkeley Longitudinal Study. In K. E. Grossmann, K. Grossmann, & E. Waters (Eds.), *Attachment from infancy to adulthood* (pp. 245–304). New York: Guilford Press.

Malchiodi, C. A. (Ed.). (2013). *Expressive therapies.* New York: Guilford Press.

Malchiodi, C. A. (2020). *Trauma and expressive arts therapy: Brain, body, and imagination in the healing process.* New York: Guilford Press.

Malchiodi, C. A., & Crenshaw, D. A. (Eds.). (2015). *Creative arts and play therapy for attachment problems.* New York: Guilford Press.

Martin, B., Jr. (1997). *Brown bear, Brown bear, what do you see?* New York: Holt.

Martin, E. E., Snow, M. S., & Sullivan, K. (2008). Patterns of relating between mothers and preschool-aged children using the Marschak Interaction Method Rating System. *Early Child Development and Care, 178*(3), 305–314.

McKinney, K. G., & Kempson, D. A. (2012). Losing touch in social work practice. *Social Work, 57*(2), 189–191.

Miller, C., & Boe, J. (1990). Tears into diamonds: Transformation of child psychic trauma through sandplay and storytelling. *Arts in Psychotherapy, 17,* 247–257.

Miller, L. J., Fuller, D. A., & Roetenberg, J. (2014). *Sensational kids: Hope and help for children with sensory processing disorder (SPD).* New York: Penguin.

Montirosso, R., Cozzi, P., Tronick, E., & Borgatti, R. (2012). Differential distribution and lateralization of infant gestures and their relation to maternal gestures in the Face-to-Face Still-Face Paradigm. *Infant Behavior and Development, 35*(4), 819–828.

Mundkur, N. (2005). Neuroplasticity in children. *Indian Journal of Pediatrics, 72,* 855–857.

Nasr, S. J. (2013). No laughing matter: Laughter is good psychiatric medicine: A case report. *Current Psychiatry, 12,* 20–25.

Newman, M. G., & Stone, A. A. (1996). Does humor moderate the effects of experimentally induced stress? *Annals of Behavioral Medicine, 18*(2), 101–109.

Nezu, A. M., Nezu, C. M., & Blissett, S. E. (1988). Sense of humor as a moderator of the relation between stressful events and psychological distress: A prospective analysis. *Social Psychology, 54,* 520–525.

Ogden, P., Minton, K., & Pain, C. (2006). *Trauma and the body: A sensorimotor approach to psychotherapy.* New York: Norton.

Otoshi, K., & Baumgarten, B. (2015). *Beautiful hands.* San Francisco: Blue Dot Press.

Overholser, J. C. (1992). Sense of humor when coping with life stress. *Personality and Individual Differences, 13,* 799–804.

Panksepp, J. (1998). Affective neuroscience: The foundation of human and animal emotion. *Consciousness and Cognition, 14,* 19–69.

Panksepp, J., & Biven, L. (2012). *The archaeology of mind: Neuroevolutionary origins of human emotions.* New York: Norton.

Payne, P., Levine, P. A., & Crane-Godreau, M. A. (2015). Somatic experiencing: Using interoception and proprioception as core elements of trauma therapy. *Frontiers in Psychology, 6,* 93.

Perry, B. D. (2000). Traumatized children: How childhood trauma influences brain development. *Journal of California Alliance for the Mentally Ill, 11*(1), 48–51.

Perry, B. D. (2006). Applying principles of neurodevelopment to clinical work with maltreated and traumatized children: The neurosequential model of therapeutics. In N. B. Webb (Ed.), *Working with traumatized youth in child welfare* (pp. 27–52). New York: Guilford Press.

Perry, B. D. (2009). Examining child maltreatment through a neurodevelopmental lens: Clinical applications of the neurosequential model of therapeutics. *Journal for Loss and Trauma, 12,* 240–255.

Pollak, S. D., Cicchetti, D., Hornung, K., & Reed, A. (2000). Recognizing emotion in faces: Developmental effects of child abuse and neglect. *Developmental Psychology, 36*(5), 679–688.

Pollak, S. D., & Sinha, P. (2002). Effects of early experience on children's recognition of facial displays of emotion. *Developmental Psychology, 38*(5), 784–791.

Porges, S. W. (2009). The polyvagal theory: New insights into adaptive reactions of the autonomic nervous system. *Cleveland Clinic Journal of Medicine, 76*(Suppl. 2), S86–S90.

Porges, S. W. (2011). *The polyvagal theory: Neurophysiological foundations of emotion, attachment, communication, and self-regulation.* New York: Norton.

Porges, S. W. (2015). Play as neural exercise: Insights from the polyvagal theory. In D. Pearce-McCall (Ed.), *The power of play for mind–brain health* (pp. 3–7). Retrieved from *https://mindgains.org/bonus/GAINS-The-Power-of-Play-for-Mind-Brain-Health.pdf.*

Powell, B., Cooper, G., Hoffman, K., & Marvin, R. (2007). The Circle of Security project: A case study—"It hurts to give that which you did not receive." In D. Oppenheim & D. F. Goldsmith (Eds.), *Attachment theory in clinical work with children: Bridging the gap between research and practice* (pp. 172–202). New York: Guilford Press.

Powell, B., Cooper, G., Hoffman, K., & Marvin, R. S. (2009). The circle of security. *Handbook of Infant Mental Health, 3,* 450–467.

Provence, S., & Lipton, R. C. (1962). *Infants in institutions.* Oxford, UK: International Universities Press.

Purvis, K., Cross, D., Dansereau, D., & Parris, S. (2013). Trust-based relational intervention (TBRI): A systemic approach to complex developmental trauma. *Child and Youth Services, 34*(4), 360–386.

Purvis, K. B., Cross, D. R., & Sunshine, W. L. (2007). *The connected child: Bring hope and healing to your adoptive family.* New York: McGraw-Hill.

Ray, D. C. (2016). *A therapist's guide to child development.* New York: Routledge.

Rose, R. (Ed.). (2017). *Innovative therapeutic life story work: Developing trauma-informed practice for working with children, adolescents and young adults.* London: Jessica Kingsley.

Rothschild, B. (2000). *The body remembers: The psychophysiology of trauma and trauma treatment.* New York: Norton.

Salters, D. (2013) Sandplay and family constellation: An integration with transactional analysis theory and practice. *Transactional Analysis Journal, 43*(3), 224–239.

Schaefer, C. E., & DiGeronimo, T. F. (2000). *Ages and stages: A parent's guide to normal childhood development.* Hoboken, NJ: Wiley.

Schore, A. N. (1996). The experience-dependent maturation of a regulatory system in the orbital prefrontal cortex and the origin of developmental psychopathology. *Development and Psychopathology, 8*(1), 59–87.

Schore, A. N. (2001). The effects of early relational trauma on right brain development, affect regulation and infant mental health. *Infant Mental Health Journal, 22*, 201–269.

Schore, A. N., & Schore, J. R. (2008). Modern attachment theory: The central role of affect regulation in development and treatment. *Clinical Social Work Journal, 39*, 9–20.

Shapiro, F. (2017). *Eye movement desensitization and reprocessing (EMDR) therapy: Basic principles, protocols, and procedures* (3rd ed.). New York: Guilford Press.

Shapiro, S. L., Carlson, L. E., Astin, J. A., & Freedman, B. (2006). Mechanisms of mindfulness. *Journal of Clinical Psychology, 62*, 373–386.

Siegel, D. J. (2010). *Mindsight: The new science of personal transformation.* New York: Bantam.

Siegel, D. J. (2020). *The developing mind* (3rd ed.). New York: Guilford Press.

Siegel, D. J., & Bryson, T. P. (2011). *The whole-brain child: 12 revolutionary strategies to nurture your child's developing mind.* New York: Bantam Books.

Siegel, D. J., & Bryson, T. P. (2018). *The yes brain: How to cultivate courage, curiosity, and resilience in your child.* New York: Bantam Books.

Siegel, D. J., & Hartzell, M. (2013). *Parenting from the inside out: How a deeper self-understanding can help you raise children who thrive.* New York: TarcherPerigee.

Sroufe, L. A., Coffino, B., & Carlson, E. A. (2010). Conceptualizing the role of early experience: Lessons from the Minnesota Longitudinal Study. *Developmental Review, 30*, 36–51.

Stein, D. E. (2009). *Pouch.* New York: Putnam.

Stewart, A. L., Field, T. A., & Echterling, L. G. (2016). Neuroscience and the magic of play therapy. *International Journal of Play Therapy, 25*(1), 4–13.

Taback, S. (2009). *This is the house that Jack built.* Charlotte, NC: Baker & Taylor

Thompson, M. R., Callaghan, P. D., Hunt G. E., Cornish, J. L., & McGregor, I. S. (2007).

A role for oxytocin and 5-HT(1A) receptors in the prosocial effects of 3,4 methylene-dioxymethamphetamine ("ecstasy"). *Neuroscience, 146*(2), 509–514.

Uvnäs-Moberg, K., & Francis, R. (2003). *The oxytocin factor: Tapping the hormone of calm, love, and healing.* Cambridge, MA: Da Capo Press.

van der Kolk, B. A. (2005). Developmental trauma disorder. *Psychiatric Annals, 35*(5), 401–408.

van der Kolk, B. A. (2015). *The body keeps the score: Brain, mind, and body in the healing of trauma.* New York: Penguin Books.

van Rosmalen, L., van der Veer, R., & van der Horst, F. (2015). Ainsworth's strange situation procedure: The origin of an instrument. *Journal of the History of the Behavioral Sciences, 51*(3), 261–284.

Verny, T. R., & Kelly, J. (1988). *The secret life of the unborn child: How you can prepare your baby for a happy, healthy life.* New York: Dell.

Vygotsky, L., & Cole, M. (1978). *Mind in society: The development of higher psychological processes.* Cambridge, MA: Harvard University Press.

Wheeler, N., & Dillman Taylor, D. (2016). Integrating interpersonal neurobiology with play therapy. *International Journal of Play Therapy, 25*(1), 24–34.

Wild, B., Rodden, F. A., Grodd, W., & Ruch, W. (2003). Neural correlates of laughter and humour. *Brain, 126*(10), 2121–2138.

Winnicott, D. W. (1953). Transitional objects and transitional phenomena—A study of the first not-me possession. *International Journal of Psychoanalysis, 34,* 84–97.

Wood, A. (2015). *The napping house.* Boston: Houghton Mifflin Harcourt.

Index

Note. The letter *f* following a page number indicates figure.

handout for, 125, 125*f*
for new experiences, 105–107
parent homework sheet for, 126*f*
Soothing
anticipatory, 61
Safe Bosses and, 60–64
self, 63
while expanding emotional literacy, 165–167, 165*f*
Static stick intervention, 185
Stealing, parental approach to, 43–45
Stick together bookmarks intervention, 186, 186*f*
Stick Together Squigz connectors, 187, 188*f*
Still Face Experiments, 64–65, 107
Stories
Delighting-In, 142, 143*f*
parental, and child's sense of self, 210–211
Storykeepers, 1, 4, 6, 8; *see also* Becoming Storykeepers
absence of, 55
parental role as, 44
Safe Boss as, 67–69
Storykeeping, parental view of behavior and, 182
Strange Situation experiments, 77–78, 106
Success, setting bar for, 45, 46*f*, 47*f*, 48
Superheroes, secret identities of, 27
SuperParents
designs for, 30*f*, 31*f*
paradigm shift and, 26–28
planning guide for, 29*f*
Sympathetic nervous system, functions of, 36

T

Tantrums, cortisol release and, 118
Therapist
and grounding in attachment theory, 77–78
as Safe Boss, 50
and secure base/safe haven training, 53
transference/countertransference and, 17
Therapist's Guide to Child Development, A (Ray), 32
There Was an Old Lady Who Swallowed a Fly (Colandro), 124
Third Ear intervention, 216–219, 216*f*
This Is the House That Jack Built (Taback), 124
Threat level, assessment of, 89, 90*f*, 91*f*, 92
Tightrope walk, 7–9
Timeline work, 55, 211–214
Timelines, garden, 234–236, 235*f*
Tone of face work, 98–100
Tone of voice, 98
Touch/physical proximity, 116–120
concerns about, 117
as regulating tool, 116–117, 119*f*
as trigger, 119–120
Toxic ruptures, 18, 20
Transference/countertransference, clinician and, 17
Transitional objects, 219–223
for connecting with absent parents, 70–71, 70*f*
Trauma
anxiety and, 67–68
brain development and, 35

reworking, 209–210
separation anxiety and, 71
TraumaPlay, 2, 4
boundary work and, 200–202
Cascade of Care and, 10
and Nurture by Proxy, 138, 139*f*
parental needs and, 5–6
training in, 79–80
Traumatized children, 35
polyvagal theory and, 35–39
Triggers
in boundary setting, 178–179, 180*f*
touch as, 119–120
Triune brain; *see also* Brain development
introducing parents to, 33–34, 33*f*
Triune brain training, 155–176
complications of, 172, 174, 175*f*, 176*f*
duality of anger and, 170–172, 171*f*, 172*f*, 173*f*
and parental development of emotional granularity and shared language, 162, 165–170, 165*f*, 170*f*
sensory processing issues and, 155–162, 163*f*, 164*f*
Tronick, Ed, 64–65, 107
Trust, development of, 58–59
"Two Choices Handouts," 108, 109*f*, 110*f*, 111

V

Vagus nerve, functions of, 35
van Eys, Patti, 93
Vanderbilt University, research project of, 93
Visual imagery, value of, 69
Voice, tone of, 98
Vygotsky, Lev, 42

W

Waze app, 121
We Are's, 214–215
Well of compassion, opening, 13–15, 16*f*
When We Stick Together Mantra, 240*f*
Window of Tolerance (WOT), 81–89
giving "yes" and, 198–199
Nurture Nook security and, 130–131
optimal arousal zone and, 86, 87*f*, 88*f*, 89
reflective exercises and, 82–89
sensory input and, 158
sensory processing and, 162
Wolchin, Rachel, 199
Worry Wars Protocol, sensory processing and, 162
WOT Are You Doing? exercise, 82–83, 83*f*
WOT Are You? exercise, 82–84, 84*f*, 85*f*, 86

Y

"Yes," giving, 197–199
Yes Brain, The (Siegel), 197